The
Psychologist's
Eat-Anything
Diet

Leonard Pearson, Ph.D.
and
Lillian Pearson, M.S.W.

with K

A Publication of The Gestalt Journal Press

Contents

PART 2
EXERCISES FOR FOOD AND DRINK
AWARENESS AND SENSUOUS EATING

Introduction to The Gestalt Journal Press Edition

This book is a gem. That it is back in print is a gift to anyone who has ever tried to lose weight, who struggles with food and eating and to those of any age who are about to head down the path for the first time.

Some of you reading this book have suffered terribly. Regardless of your size — you diet, you overeat, you try, you quit, you lose, you gain.

Leonard and Lillian Pearson, a psychologist and social worker who worked with eating problems for more than twenty years, understand *you*; and this book addresses *all* your issues with a comprehensive approach to eating and losing weight.

The Pearsons' explanation of the cause of the problem is straightforward — dieting and the "diet mentality" backfire. Using easily understood ideas and examples from everyday situations, the Pearsons offer new ways to approach food and eating in your life — minimizing deprivation and maximizing satisfaction — freeing you from food demons and food police. While reading the book, you explore the personal dimensions of your hungers and appetites. You increase your self/food awareness. You explore a variety of eating "situations" (lunch with colleagues, dinner with friends, holidays with relatives, nighttime snacks, etc.) and are encouraged to find *your* best method for handling them. You are given tools — not rules.

"O.K." you say, "but how do I lose weight?" As you learn how to decrease deprivation and increase satisfaction you take in less food. Your cravings, your "hunger," your over-eating — diminish.

Read this book. Even better, read it with a friend or two and work with it together. Read it again — a chapter here, a chapter there. New ideas need time to digest. New approaches take practice.

For many years in my private practice, I counseled people with eating problems. Too fat, too thin — starvers, stuffers, chronic dieters — children and adults, men and women. It would surprise you to learn how many things they have in common — despite what they look like on the outside. This book gave something to every single one of them.

The Psychologists Eat Anything Diet gives readers two great gifts: *Forgiveness* and *hope*. It's not your fault — and there is a "way out." Whether you use all the book or just parts of it — in your world of eating you'll be better equipped, happier with yourself, and more at peace with food.

Molly Rawle M.S.W.
Director — The River Center for the Study of Eating Disorders

PART 1

THE PSYCHOLOGY OF OVEREATING

1/ *WHERE ITS AT*

This is a book about food liberation.

We have a radical approach to the problems of overeating and overweight. It is based on insights gained in seventeen years of successful clinical practice in Chicago, Cleveland, and currently, at The Pearson Institute in Berkeley, California. Our purely psychological way of dealing with these problems has been successful in the overwhelming majority of cases. This is in marked contrast to the extremely poor success rate of more traditional methods and dieting by pills, which are shown to have a long term success rate of only 2 percent, according to recent reliable scientific studies.

When you have finished this book, you should be able to:

❏   Eat your favorite foods.
❏   Realize that there are no forbidden foods and taboos.
❏   Free yourself and your entire family from the tyranny of food.
❏   Pleasure yourself with food and drink.
❏   Donate your scales to the Salvation Army.
❏   Throw away your calorie charts and diet lists.
❏   Forget about proteins, carbohydrates, fats and all the other old diet standbys.

Guilt feelings, regimentation, and deprivation have no place in our method. We will show how permanent weight loss can take place in an atmosphere of freedom. Even though it may sound like an impossible dream — such as the repeal of income taxes — it is a fact: the foods you crave and love are the ones you should eat. Hunger has many causes, and we will help you find them.

We believe that restrictive weight-losing schemes — such as Weight Watchers' — are based on archaic ideas. We think it is dead wrong to do battle with yourself. Reliance on old standbys like willpower, self-denial, discipline, and self-control leads to a state of inner warfare that is psychologically damaging. In addition, these dietary regimes rarely lead to permanent solutions.

We will demonstrate clear-cut ways to heighten awareness of food and of the eating process; to increase the efficiency of appetite satisfaction; and to lead the reader toward an understanding of the personal needs that are served by overeating. Our ultimate goal is to guide the reader toward a permanent, secure weight loss in an atmosphere of freedom.

On the surface, the ideas of pleasuring yourself with food and simultaneously losing weight do seem incompatible. But they are not — once you've gotten your signals straight, once you understand what food and eating — to you very personally — are really all about.

Overeating is a complex process and has many causes. We will offer exercises for developing insights into this complex process. But first things first: We have found that one of the most common causes is that people don't eat enough of what they love and crave. Their eating, restricted by diet advice and orientation toward calorie-counting, gives them little satisfaction. So they must eat more. And then some more.

Psychologically speaking, eating must give satisfaction. Otherwise, it is inefficient and wasteful. Many people eat through a filter of guilt and ambivalence. This interferes with getting emotional satisfaction from food. It's best to give yourself permission to eat whatever you like — and forever. Then, along with this permission, you need to develop insights and food awareness.

To help you begin creating food awareness, we want to introduce a concept basic to our method. We call it "humming and beckoning."

Foods that "hum" to you are those that you really crave and love — quite regardless of immediate availability.

Foods that "beckon" to you are those that you had not been craving. It is a food that's available now. "It looks good," "it will taste fine," it starts to appeal to you, to invite you.

When a certain food hums to you, you yearn for it. When a food beckons, it calls out to you. They are two distinct, quite different events.

The image of humming derives from its similarity to a tune that you can't get out of your head. Foods that hum can almost be heard inside your head. It's as if a message is coming up from inner depths, directing you toward a particular food, persisting until you respond.

Beckoning foods aren't on your mind. Quite often, even the idea of eating isn't on your mind — until you look in that bakery window, get a whiff from that candy kitchen, or notice delicious-looking food being served at the next table.

It is important, at the outset, to distinguish between these two situations.

Not that there is anything wrong with eating food that beckons to you. But if you don't follow your craving, if you don't eat the food that hums and eat a beckoning food *instead*, you will not feel satisfied.

You may still feel hungry.

When foods hum to you, you can almost literally taste them, smell them, feel them. We believe that these are the foods you should eat. Eat them *when* you want them, *where* you want them, and as *much* of them as you feel like.

To summarize the differences between humming and beckoning:

Humming Food	*Beckoning Food*
1. You think of the food without seeing it, or before seeing it.	1. This food wasn't on your mind until you saw it.
2. You yearn for the food.	2. The food calls out to you.
3. The food may not even be immediately available.	3. The food is immediately available.
4. A food you feel a craving for, right now. Desire for the food comes from inner depths.	4. It looks good. You'd enjoy it, but you don't crave it.
5. It satisfies "hunger."	5. It tastes good but doesn't satisfy. Or you have to overeat to get the satisfaction of fullness.

What about calories? This issue is usually useless and destructive. It focuses attention solely on presumed weight loss and tunes out what your food desires are. Calorie-counting perpetuates a state of futile warfare within yourself. And that does not lead to *permanent* weight loss.

What's more, the calorie games played by many so-called diet and nutrition experts are illogical and even bizarre. Let's look at just one. Recently, one "expert" made headlines by announcing that sex is the answer to obesity. His peerless reasoning was that you burn up about 300 calories making love. What's more, during the time you spend in bed with your partner, you aren't eating food — thus saving even more calories. Therefore, by having intercourse three times weekly you could lose four pounds a month.

In the first place, it is patent nonsense to talk of how many calories you burn up during intercourse. A glance at the Masters and Johnson research (or even just the porno comic books at the neighborhood cigar stand) indicates that human sexual contact has infinite variety. The amount of time people spend and the positions they assume during the sex act are just two of many variables. To talk of any average amount of energy — or calories — is naive.

In addition, it's a false assumption that, if you don't opt for sex, you'd spend your time snacking. Finally, we know many people who pleasure themselves with food before, during, or after the sex act.

This entire scheme might be shrugged off if it didn't have some definitely unhealthy implications. It advocates an exploitive use of sex. Sex for a calorie loss is fundamentally the same as sex for pay: It totally corrupts a rewarding and powerful human experience and turns it into prescribed medicine to help you lose weight!

We have observed how the same thing happens at times with outdoor sports. When people swim or play tennis as part of a reducing scheme, the joy and spirit tend to go out of the sport. Instead of providing vigor, relaxation, and a sense of one's body movements, the sport becomes still another chore, one more thing you must make yourself do to help you lose weight.

Has this happened to you? And how many years have you been counting calories? What has it done for you?

Not much, according to most people we work with. They have lost and gained, lost and gained, and then gained some more. Many say, grimly, "I've lost one thousand pounds in fifteen years, and gained one thousand twenty." Still, many people tend to cling to calorie-counting, because "If I didn't watch my calories, I'd gain a hundred pounds." People greatly fear the idea of deviating from an established pattern, even one that has been an unmitigated failure.

You may have wondered about the secret of slender people who never diet. You have probably thought that some of your thin friends are being coy when someone asks them, "How do you stay so thin?" and they answer, "I don't know, I just eat what I feel like." Actually, their answer is quite sensible. They are so free that they are not even aware of their liberated relationship to food. It would never occur to them to eat something they didn't want or to eat when they didn't desire food. (Obviously, we're not referring to "thinnies" who are constantly doing battle with food and dieting desperately.)

GO AHEAD: EAT THREE ECLAIRS

Suppose what really hums to you is a chocolate eclair from your best local pastry shop. Lots of calories? Certainly. But suppose you eat that eclair; no, let's suppose you eat not one but three of them this afternoon. If you eat them without thinking of the calories, without feeling the guilt of having fallen off the wagon, it will be a delightful, satisfying experience. So satisfying, in fact, that the steak, green beans, and tossed salad with low-calorie dressing that you had planned for dinner may not hum to you at all. So don't eat them. *The freedom to eat will also give you the freedom to not eat.*

We want to stress that there is a great distinction between skipping dinner because you feel you have been bad and want to save on calories, and skipping dinner because you feel satisfied and have no real desire to eat. The first is a form of punishment, something you impose upon yourself and your body — a deprivation. The second is living by the wisdom of your body, tuning into yourself and following the signals that you receive from nature.

And since we assume that calories are still on your mind, let's point out that the eclairs contain about the same number of calories as the steak-vegetable-and-salad dinner. By caloric count, you'd be even. However, from a psychological viewpoint you would be more satisfied and more in harmony with yourself.

Consider the eclairs a little further. If you sit at your desk, close your eyes, and out of nowhere (seemingly) come the taste, smell, and texture of an eclair — if you can practically feel the slightly sticky bitter-sweetness of the chocolate icing, the airy texture of the dough that gives just a little resistance to your teeth, and then the utterly lickable soft creaminess of the filling — then the eclair is humming to you. By contrast, if you walk down the street, happen to look into the bakery shop window, see a platter of eclairs, and think, "Wouldn't that be great?" that isn't humming, that's beckoning.

To yield to such beckoning foods can interfere with really tuning into yourself; it's settling for second best when only the best is really good enough for you.

In practical terms, yielding to beckoning foods easily leads to overeating. The process goes something like this: A food is beckoning, so you buy some (or get it out of the refrigerator) and eat it. But it isn't quite what you wanted (what hummed), so then something else beckons, and you eat that in hopes that it will do the job. You still have that vague feeling (I'm hungry for something) and hope that the second food will satisfy you. But it doesn't. Nor does food number three, or four, or five. By that time, you may feel slightly bloated, and you are probably building up intense guilt feelings for eating more than is good for you, more than you wanted. The real trouble is that you have not eaten anything that is good for you in the sense of meeting your psychological needs.

It is not easy to learn to distinguish between foods that hum and foods that beckon, particularly if you have been spending many years fighting against yourself, trying to ignore and blank out the signals from within.

We worked with one man, a thirty-eight-year-old, 288-pound accountant of Greek ancestry, who loved pilaff. Pilaff often hummed to him, but he never allowed himself to eat it because, he reasoned, rice is heavy in carbohydrates and, furthermore, in pilaff the rice is sauteed in butter. He wanted to consume fewer calories and lower his cholesterol count.

He ate lunch every day at a smorgasbord restaurant near his office, and every day he would virtuously bypass the pilaff. What he would end up eating were portions of chicken equivalent to two or three whole chickens!

This, in our experience, is quite typical. The person who denies himself the food that hums will start eating "around" what he really wants and end up consuming far more calories than the forbidden food contains.

> We have found that there is one uncomplicated way of ascertaining what hums — what you really want: Ask yourself, *"Will I feel cheated if I don't get this?"*

If it really hums, you'll feel cheated by any substitute, no matter how delicious and tempting (beckoning) it might be.

We have checked out this test over the years, and it seems to be a nearly foolproof method.

HOW TO TELL IF IT'S HUMMING

Two examples — one positive, one negative — demonstrate our method as well as the pitfalls to avoid.

A professional couple attending one of our Institute's occasional out-of-town obesity workshops — this one in Reno, Nevada — had some business to attend to after the session was over at 5:00 P.M. By the time this appointment was finished, they both felt ravenously hungry.

The wife, Kim,[*] had a strong craving for eggs with hash-brown potatoes. Her husband, Ken, wanted a big, fine steak. They decided on a top restaurant about which they had heard, partly because they wanted to conclude the evening in a pleasant atmosphere and also because they figured they might not come to Reno again for a long time. (The notion of eating some place new when traveling, because "we'll never be here again," is a common one, and can exaggerate the extent of your hunger. Try to order just what you feel like — a drink, or just dessert — and enjoy the atmosphere.)

Before they had even opened their menu, Kim watched with fascination as a most unusual salad was prepared for a couple at the next table. It contained all sorts of superbly crisp-looking greens, but what intrigued her most were chunks of fresh pineapple and succulent crab legs.

She wavered on her decision about eggs and hash browns, telling herself (among other things) that you can eat eggs and hash browns anytime, in any roadside restaurant, but you could not get this kind of salad.

Then Ken told her which steak on the menu he had chosen — a filet served with Bearnaise sauce and trimmings. Suddenly, that too sounded tempting. To make matters even worse, she saw "club sandwich de luxe" listed on the menu; club sandwich is another of her favorites.

---

[*]All names, places of residence, and other identifying data in this book have been altered to protect the privacy of the people involved.

All these foods beckoned; all, Kim was sure, would be delicious, appealingly served, and totally enjoyable. What should she do?

She finally put down the menu, closed her eyes, and asked herself, "Will I feel cheated if I don't get that salad?" She decided the answer was "no."

She went on to examine whether she would feel cheated watching Ken eat that steak and not having one herself. The answer again was "no." The same was true of the club sandwich. But when she came to eggs and hash browns, she felt a clear inner "yes." She definitely would feel cheated without this one dish. And so she ordered it from a slightly surprised French waiter and enjoyed it thoroughly. Even though this was the only food she had had in ten hours, she had no inclination to eat dessert. She had eaten what hummed to her, and was totally satisfied.

The very opposite happened to Barbara, an energetic, forty-four-year-old business executive. She had gone to several "fat farms" to try and lose her twenty-pound excess. Prior to coming to a workshop at our Institute in Berkeley, she said, she had been losing the same twenty pounds for almost two decades.

At the end of the first session, Friday evening, when all participants are encouraged to go out and eat what really hums to them, she didn't hesitate one moment: She wanted Monterey Abalone with a baked potato and sour cream and chives dressing. She went to a nearby fish restaurant. She ordered her abalone and baked potato. She ignored the salad and French bread the waiter brought to the table first.

Then came the abalone — with French-fried potatoes. It wasn't the baked potato she had envisioned. The waiter told her that abalone came with French fries. "I didn't think it would matter. I like French fries, and I never allow myself to eat them at home. So I decided, what's the difference, I might as well eat the fries."

The trouble is that there *was* a difference, and when we discussed it the next day she realized that she did feel disappointed and a little cheated because she hadn't gotten her baked potato — so much so that after the French fries she had also polished off the salad and French bread plus two desserts.

Plainly, the French fries beckoned. The baked potato had hummed, and therefore would have been the right food for Barbara.

The ability to discern humming from beckoning food is one of the components leading to food satisfaction and liberated eating. This can be a new lifestyle for you that leads to natural and permanent weight loss.

In order to learn what foods hum to you, you have to throw away exchange lists and diet lists of forbidden, taboo, "poison," and "illicit" foods. You have to take *all* foods out of quarantine. That also means taking yourself out of the prison of dieting.

2/ DIETS ARE JAILS UNFIT
FOR HUMAN BEINGS

This chapter is about people who spend their lives dieting — or feeling that they should be dieting. These two feelings can ruin your lifestyle, because guilt and enjoyment make poor bedfellows. Many people with eating problems are so laden with guilt feelings that they dilute the pleasure available from food.

They find themselves in a bind. They love eating, but they hate what food "does to them." They dislike, even detest, the size of their own body. And they believe that they weigh too much because they eat too much.

This assumption is generally correct. According to the American Medical Association, of the approximately sixty million Americans who are obese, only 5 percent suffer from any metabolic malfunction or endocrine disorder. The rest overeat.

In attempts to solve overeating, traditional diets and weight-losing schemes advocate that you fight back against food by rigid regimentation.

Many people we have worked with over the years have shared one image: They think of themselves as being imprisoned forever by diet dictators. They are in a jail whenever they diet (and on parole between periods of dieting). All the delicious, enjoyable food in the world is just outside the prison walls, but the cops keep twenty-four-hour guard and won't let the prisoners out or let any of that wonderful food in. Depending on the individual, the cops may be diets, doctors, admonitions, threats, fear of the scales, or fear of guilt feelings, friends, or family members.

Every so often, the generally docile prisoner rebels; he or she has had all he can take. There is a jail break. The prisoner then gets out into that wonderful world of food, throws all rules and restrictions to the wind, and gorges. Not seeing any road out of this predicament except through that grim jailhouse, he eats more and more, promising "just this time and never again; tomorrow I'll start dieting seriously."

It is an experience in ambivalence. Guilt and shame get in the way, filtering out much of the pleasure.

This does not mean that in a short while the person will stop eating and dutifully return to the diet jail. Another part of the guilt syndrome comes into play. There is that awful feeling that since you did disrupt the regimen, since you did fall off the wagon, you have blown it for the day, maybe even the week. You've demonstrated how inadequate and incompetent you are as a human being.

Many obese people tell how after a jail break they have continued eating and gorging the rest of the day or week — or even a month during the Christmas season. But they did so, feeling guilty and dissatisfied, feeling "once again I have failed." In such an atmosphere of guilt and futility, nobody can find much food satisfaction.

To most people, binging represents the ultimate fall from grace. You may sneak some candy or ice cream or cheese or nuts and tell yourself that you will make up for it by not eating bread or potatoes at dinner. But there is no excuse, no making up for the binge — only feelings of self-hate, anger, disappointment, and discouragement.

Binging, almost needless to say, usually involves forbidden foods that are high in calories, very often in what establishment nutritionists glibly label "empty calories." Almost nobody binges on celery sticks. We have found that chocolate, whether in candy, ice cream, or cake, is very often involved in binging. But for some people it might be pecan pie, or sundaes, or potato chips, or spaghetti. The list can be long and diversified.

For some people binges mean "I'll eat anything if it doesn't move." They also lament that they behave like a vacuum cleaner.

CONFESSIONS OF A BINGE EATER

"I hate myself when I am binging, and I cannot look at myself when it's over," related Helen, the thirty-two-year-old wife of a dentist. She binges on sweets, especially pies, when the children are in school and her husband is at work.

"When I start a binge, I tell myself I'm just going to have a little candy. I buy half a dozen candy bars and tell myself that I'll only eat one and give the rest to the children. But I eat them all. Then I decide that I'll never do this again, that this is the last time. And I go out and get several pies, each one at a different bakery. I drive far enough away from home so they won't know me. And even then I always give the clerk an explanation and say something about a party.

"I feel I have to make up excuses, even for strangers, but I always have a terrible feeling that they don't believe me anyway. I think they look at me and say to themselves, 'Look at that fat cow; I bet she eats it all herself.' And, of course, I do. I eat till I am physically ill. That usually happens halfway through the last pie, Then I flush the rest down the disposal and burn the boxes, so the kids won't suspect."

It's fairly evident that binging brings little pleasure — especially afterward.

We have found that the person who never feels imprisoned in his eating has little desire to start the kind of prison riot that a binge represents. There is no need to. In the case of Helen, if she allowed herself to eat pie whenever she felt like it, as much as she felt like, with full sensory awareness, but *only* when she felt like it, she would not have to binge. The pies are "out there" forever. They are always available. They need not only be consumed when the coast is clear. That is an external signal.

But when you have the feeling that tomorrow the jailers will be back in power, maybe forever after, the binge becomes a necessity for emotional survival. No human being can live with so bleak a prospect as never again being allowed to do (or eat) what he wants. In this way the binging does have psychological value — it is an assertion of basic rights and a rejection of enslavement. In other words, it is a healthy response to dietary deprivation.

One newcomer to our Institute, a late-fortyish divorced teacher, carrying 190 pounds on a basically slender five-foot-five frame and as concerned about her looks and her chances for a second marriage as she was about her health, asked incredulously: "You mean to tell me I should actually buy a banana split and *enjoy* it? I thought our objective here was to lose weight, not lose the few inhibitions we have about food. If I lose my inhibitions, I'll become mountainous!"

In other words, she clung to jail as her salvation, and the thought of pleasuring herself with food seemed sinful. Yet, her reliance on inhibitions had failed her for years.

Much later, she came to see that there is no inconsistency between losing weight and enjoying the pleasures of food. If anything, they are positively correlated. As we explored her overeating patterns, she found alternatives and also developed greater awareness of food sensations. Finally she formed a new relationship to food. Her weight loss has not been spectacular, but it has been steady (a pound every week for the past seven months), and she feels free about her body and her eating. Overeating had never given her any pleasure; now, eating does.

3/ *THE PUT-DOWN SOCIETY AND YOUR VIEW OF YOUR SELF*

This chapter deals with people who mistakenly blame their weight problem on lack of willpower, poor self-control, or similar psychological defects. It should also help people, particularly women, who forever chase a dream of an ideal weight and a perfect figure.

People with weight or eating problems are frequently labeled-by others or by themselves — "compulsive eaters," "oral personalities," "oral-dependent personalities," or "nocturnal hyperphagic" (which merely means "someone who eats a lot at night" but sounds like an expensive pathological condition).

All these terms have a pseudoscientific ring to them. The trouble is that they are nothing but empty phrases. Some of the dozens, if not hundreds, of clichés freely attached to overeaters.

If you were to believe everything you read, then the following people would have to be classified as "oral personalities" or "oral-dependent personalities":

- People who eat too much (at least sixty million people in the U.S.).

- People who smoke (according to available statistics, 24 percent of our adult population, or over fifty million).
- People who drink alcohol in excess (nine million).
- People who are addicted to non-alcoholic drinks (Coke, 7-Up, ice water, or rose hip tea qualify, and who could count all the addicts?).
- People who talk too much.

No statistics are available on the last two categories, but if you add them all up, almost all people in the country are "oral-dependent personalities." In other words, the term is scientifically meaningless!

We urge people to reexamine labels such as "poor will-power" and "oral personality." There is a sound basis for questioning the validity of such negative labels. There is also good reason to reject the whole idea of labeling oneself.

There has been an unfortunate tendency in the last few years for people to attach all kinds of labels to themselves as a way of "psyching out" the self. We say this is unfortunate because this lay analysis does little good — and much harm. To psychologize with labels achieves the very opposite of its desired aims: It creates a distance between you and your feelings; it divides rather than unifies; it creates a false entity, a dichotomy within yourself.

If you label yourself an "oral personality" then you have created an artificial distance between you and your behavior. You have pigeonholed and classified an aspect of yourself. You have computerized certain behavior into a generalized concept called "orality." This interferes with exploring, experiencing, and becoming more aware of yourself. It's a meaningless process of searching for pathological labels for common behavior. It stops the process of growth. A label can stagnate self-understanding. (It's ironic that we don't feel a need to classify or label behavior that is joyful or acceptable, events that go with happiness or comfort.)

Here are examples of some labels we frequently hear at our Institute:

"I have a dependency problem related to my eating."

"I stuff myself with food to compensate for my fear of abandonment."

"I love milk, cottage cheese, and yoghurt because they're all mother's-milk-type food; I'm an oral-dependent personality."

"I am a masochist and eat to punish myself."

HOW LABELS HURT

In some instances, these statements might have historical accuracy. But labeling oneself, seeing oneself as part of a psychological category, is highly unsuccessful in terms of *changing behavior*. It makes weight loss much harder, if not impossible. For example, the man who said he loved cottage cheese sometimes ate four to five pounds a day, feeling sure it was symbolic of his dependency on Mother. During the workshop he had a fantasy that he was drowning in milk — with the realization that he didn't even like it!

Let us suggest that the next time someone, whether layman or expert, labels you "oral-dependent," you might counter with a few questions of your own. For example:

"You still smoke, I see!"

"This is your third cup of coffee this morning, isn't it?"

"How many packs of gum do you go through in a day?"

"You enjoy talking, don't you?"

Thoughtful label-dispensers will stop to reexamine their labeling habit. Those who take offense because they labeled you "for your own good" are no loss. They are part of the excess baggage the obese tend to lug around in addition to their excess poundage.

Often, overweight persons don't feel free to openly reject such "helpful" comments, yet soon afterward they have to eat — eat even more than usual in many instances — to comfort and reassure themselves and assert their autonomy.

Another label put on people who overeat is that they are weak-willed or totally lacking in willpower. That, too, doesn't stand up under close scrutiny.

For a simple but indisputable start: A great many high achievers, people who are at the very top of their profession or calling, are also overweight. Secondly, obese people very often display considerable willpower in obtaining the foods they want. One of our most graphic examples was provided by Nancy, who came to our Institute a year ago.

NO WILLPOWER?

She was in her mid-thirties, extremely well groomed and attractive, but about thirty pounds over what she thought she should weigh. She was a tenured teacher.

She had recently taken her first trip to Europe, the high point of which was a visit to her father's native village in Norway, where she had aunts and cousins she had never seen.

They got along famously. One morning, talking of food, she mentioned that her favorite of all favorites was pizza. "Pizza, what's that?" said the Norwegian cousins.

Nancy was appalled that they had never even sampled this delicacy and said, "I'll make it for you for supper."

She had made pizza many times before, so this did not seem a rash statement. But she had not figured on the limitations of a Norwegian village grocery. There was cheese in abundance, but no cheese suitable for pizza, nor the right salami, not to mention fresh mushrooms, which to Nancy were essential. Even the ingredients for her kind of tomato sauce weren't all available.

Before the day was out, Nancy had caught a train to the nearby large town, from which she took a jet to Rome, shopped there for mozzarella cheese, salami, etc., and flew back in time to catch the late afternoon commuter train. At a slightly late supper, the Norwegian cousins had their first pizza.

You might call this eccentric behavior; you might call it frivolous or wasteful; but weak-willed? Hardly.

We also know of a career woman who used to drive thirty miles after a full business day for a certain kind of ice cream; an intern who, having worked a night shift, would get up after only three hours' sleep to be at his favorite bakery when the "bear-claws" arrived hot from the oven; and a Dallas executive who juggled a complicated business schedule just so he could be in New York on a day when Etinger's made blackout cake!

All these stories contain an element of the unusual. The people involved are usually the first to admit that. But whatever else anybody might say about them, these overweight people could hardly be accused of lacking willpower or determination. They expended an enormous amount of energy to plan and carry out the achievement of their particular food goal. They expressed a *strong will toward food*.

NO MORE DIETARY PURITANISM

Our country is being subjected to an intensified wave of "dietary puritanism." This is in strange contrast to the "sexual revolution," where almost everything sexual goes; yet we are expected to deny ourselves food. Likewise, the business man who works fifteen hours a day and has had at least one coronary is usually called "strong-willed," "goal-oriented," or "determined." No one would think of calling him "lacking in willpower," even though he is undermining his health as much, or more, than an obese person. He is "yielding to work," but since the end result is socially approved, the labels are more approving than those attached to the obese.

Let us make it clear: We are not propagandizing that overweight is attractive, or that fat is beautiful. This book *is* aimed at helping you *lose* weight, but self-hate does not help.

Not only do some people look at an overweight individual with suspicion and prejudice, but that person comes to internalize this low view and is expected to look on himself or herself as a second-class citizen.

The very people who consider themselves their champions — the diet advocates, founders of clubs for the obese, etc. — are usually among their worst persecutors, demanding that the overweight start from the premise that they are not quite the equals of their slender fellow citizens.

Every obese person has run into situations where a job, or a promotion, or some social nicety was withheld because he or she is overweight. The reasoning goes something like this: If this person doesn't have the willpower and self-respect to manage and control his own body, there is something wrong and he is not to be trusted because he is likely to be undisciplined and weak-willed, regardless of any data to the contrary. Obviously, this is not the kind of person to entrust with responsibility, or, indeed, to associate with too closely.

We are impressed with how obese people are mistreated by society, and how the equation seems to be: Overweight = lack of control = unworthy human being. Even though no brain structure exists for "food willpower," and new findings in humanistic psychology tell us that concepts like "willpower" and "self-control" are now obsolete in explaining human behavior, society's censure still persists.

We want to reemphasize the saddest aspect of this propaganda: Overweight people are expected to accept this view — and very often do.

Many others suffer from low self-esteem because their bodies are out of line with society's ideal. In our work we encounter many people who are aware of their own worth and their positive attributes, but they view these as secondary. These talents and qualities are overshadowed, if not blotted out, by an "imperfect" body. This is especially true with women.

The American model of physical beauty is ridiculously dictatorial. Many people we have worked with are no more than ten or eight or maybe only five pounds over their theoretically correct body weight. Some are right on the mark. Yet somehow their body measurements and proportions don't add up to the American dream of the "perfect body."

The person with this "imperfect" body, particularly if female and overweight, is urged to (and frequently feels obliged to) hide that body in something resembling a sack: shapeless suits, "unobtrusive" dresses, voluminous sweaters, and tent-like coats (the latter to be worn practically all the time). In addition, she seeks refuge in camouflage colors such as gray, brown, and black.

Whatever merits there may be in the dispute over male chauvinism in American society, it cannot be denied that a double standard operates when it comes to body perfection (or imperfection). Physical flaws, deviations from the "perfect body," are more readily accepted or overlooked in a male. And even when imperfection is acknowledged, there is far less tendency to judge a man's whole person on the basis of his body. His professional achievements, intelligence, humor, his standing in the community, even his bankbook, get strong consideration. Therefore, his self-image is not as likely to be damaged by obesity as a woman's is.

In the case of a woman, even if in fact men seem to be attracted to her, it is hard to think of herself as sexy. A woman's total worth is frequently assessed by her looks. For her, it often outweighs all other attributes if there is a flaw in her figure.

Parenthetically, it is interesting that even the term "figure" is rarely applied to the male. He is of heavy "build," has a strong "physique," a large "frame," is built "squarely" or "athletically." When the word "figure" is used for the over-weight male, it is still in a rather complimentary or at least conciliatory way, as in "portly figure."

Militant champions of women's rights say that the American woman is treated as a sex object, and there is ample evidence of that view. But how do most heavy women treat *themselves*? There is no question that the tape measure and the bathroom scales can be their daily judgment and undoing. How often have you let these devices set your mood and determine your value for the whole day?

TRYING TO CONQUER YOURSELF MAKES NO SENSE

This is another point on which we radically differ with the establishment approach toward overweight. Diet advocates and weight-reducing groups generally operate on the assumption that you must conquer part of yourself, that you have to subdue and obliterate that part of your personality assumed to be responsible for your overeating.

This presupposes that part of you isn't legitimate and that you should slice it off like a surgeon removes a wart.

This is naive and unworkable. Rather than battle a-gainst yourself and deny part of yourself the right to exist, you need to *explore* and affirm yourself. That is the beginning of the road to freedom and a weight loss that will be more than a seesaw game with the scales.

4/ *THE PSYCHOLOGY OF HUNGER: A NEW VIEW*

This is about people who frequently feel full, yet crave more food — and those who eat when they're not physically hungry. We deal with the use of food for soothing, comforting, or rewarding oneself and show how different kinds of hunger are related to specific food cravings.

"I'm hungry."

On the surface that would appear to be one of the simplest statements in any language. It is actually a very complicated statement, a loaded one, because it covers a wide variety of human experiences, sensations, reactions, and needs.

Hunger is simple only when it is a life-or-death matter. In recent years the peoples of Bangladesh and Biafra experienced a hunger that was unequivocal. It was a hunger that foreshadowed death; food, any food, meant hope of life. That is terrible, elemental, and simple hunger.

But when most of us in the rest of the world say, "I'm hungry," or even when we say, "I'm starving," we are a long way from physical damage, let alone death or dying.

"Hunger," as we customarily use the word, describes an extremely complex chain of events in humans. And exploring what hunger means to you personally is essential in trying to establish a new relationship to food, to eating, and to find alternatives to overeating.

We have found several identifiable components of that deceptive state called "being hungry."

- One element is the *locale* or site where hunger or food craving is experienced, either in the alimentary canal (stomach, throat, teeth, tongue, lips) or through hunger *head*aches, *stomach*aches or *chest* pains, to name a few.
- Another aspect is the type of food sensation, texture or quality that is sought (soft and creamy, brittle and salty, warm and starchy, etc.).
- Another element is the *psychological* category the food falls into (reward, security, cultural-ethnic).
- The last component is the emotional trigger, or precipitant, of eating, such as anger, boredom, tension, and so on.

Suppose a person feels hurt or disappointed or bored or lonely. He or she wants to be psychologically comforted or soothed, and there is usually no direct way. Since the emotional body-need of unexpressed feeling still exists, it is then often translated into a craving or hunger in a part of the alimentary canal. The craving is frequently for a texture or sensation that can be best satisfied by a particular food. If the person is tuned into this process, the result is eating a food that hums and will satisfy the craving efficiently and with pleasure.

We want to amplify each part of this process so you can observe it occurring within yourself and satisfy it in the most effective and pleasurable way. To anchor this discussion on the element that each person is most familiar with, we will begin with a discussion of the *locale of hunger*.

The most common place where hunger or craving for food is felt is in the pit of the stomach, usually as an emptiness or gnawing sensation in the gut. This is true for many people, but by no means all. Though the hunger sensation is usually experienced somewhere within the alimentary canal, it is felt outside of it by some. To determine where you experience what you call hunger is important knowledge about yourself; it can yield vital clues to your eating or overeating patterns. If you know the location and quality of your hunger, you can seek out the best sensation to satisfy yourself. *Often people are searching for a sensation rather than a food.*

PHYSIOLOGICAL VERSUS PSYCHOLOGICAL HUNGER

True physiological hunger is fairly easy to identify: It is almost always felt as hunger pangs — definite contractions of the stomach. It is also fairly simple to satisfy. A few bites of food will generally stop hunger pangs. One third of a banana, for example, is generally sufficient. The important point is: a *small* quantity of almost *any* food will suffice.

Physiological hunger thereby differs radically from the psychological kind of hunger (or food-craving) that most concerns us here. The latter is rarely satisfied by a few bites and definitely cannot be satisfied by just any food.

We want to discuss these hunger sites in detail as a means of aiding you in identifying them in the future. In addition to the common sites of hunger to be described below, we have worked with people who found, under close scrutiny, that they overate when they felt "hunger" in their shoulders, in their chest or heart or buttocks, or when they had "hunger headaches" or were aching for food throughout their body. One person at a workshop experienced hunger as a stabbing pain between her shoulder blades. During the weekend we found that in her relationships with people she tends to set herself up to be stabbed in the back and then feels ravenously hungry afterward to comfort herself.

Let us look at the four most common locales. Incidentally, these four need not be mutually exclusive. Frequently, two or more can be involved at the same time, or a person may experience hunger at different sites at different times, depending on mood and circumstances.

I. STOMACH HUNGER

Hunger experienced in the pit of the stomach may be a sensation of emptiness or of a bottomless pit, or a gnawing, or disturbing feeling in the stomach area, or an awareness of the beginnings of emptiness. It can be deceptively similar to true physiological hunger.

But the stomach hunger we are discussing is a feeling of emptiness rather than a contraction. This kind of hunger is generally satisfied by large quantities of food, and often only by something soothing and warm. When people experience this hunger sensation they sometimes "shovel it in," or "wolf it down," "inhale it," or "vacuum it" — "it" being almost any food that happens to be handy. Others keep snacking and munching all evening. No matter how large the quantity, though — and some eat to the stage of feeling bloated, uncomfortable, sick or in pain — they may remain unsatisfied if they don't eat the right food.

By "right" we do not refer to calories or carbohydrate content, or any other nutritional evaluation. We mean food that is psychologically right, food that hums. To most people with a pit-of-the-stomach-hunger feeling, what usually hums are foods with bulk, or warm, filling foods, often starchy.

If you fall into this category, try checking it out. What hums? Fresh bread, spaghetti, potatoes, rice, hominy, thick pea soup?

Many people with this hunger feeling never have a satisfying eating experience because all the foods they crave are forbidden; they are usually high in calories and carbohydrates. So what happens?

We worked with one secretary who described it well. "I always keep plenty of rabbit food in the refrigerator so I can nibble without getting any calories. So when I get this terrible hunger feeling, I start on the celery and carrots. I usually eat the whole bowl, but it doesn't do much good. Then I'll start on the cottage cheese, and I usually finish the whole container.

"Then the hunt really begins, because I'm still hungry and have eaten all the low-calorie stuff. Oh, if I have tomatoes in the house I slice them to go with the cottage cheese. Then I'll open a can of fruit or two, and maybe some tuna that's packed in water.

"I try to keep a bare kitchen, so unless I've bought stuff for guests, I have to go out at that point, because even if there are things I could cook, like meat, I can't be bothered. That would take too long.

"There is a hamburger stand nearby, and that's where I usually go. I tell them I have company at my place and order four hamburgers and milkshakes to go. I start eating the hamburgers in the car.

"I have also gone to a Colonel Sanders Shop and gotten a bucket of fried chicken and biscuits, but that isn't quite as good as the hamburgers."

The secretary later came to realize that what really satisfied her most of all were the buns. Soft bread really hums to her. Instead of rabbit food, she vows keeps several kinds of bread in the cupboard and a couple of loaves of white, rye, and wholewheat bread in the freezer, along with a dozen hamburger buns. When she gets hungry, she puts a whole loaf into a basket and sets out a pretty placemat and plate, plus a glass of wine.

She then sits down and starts eating bread, savoring it deliberately with enjoyment and gusto. She eats as much as she wants and keeps reassuring herself that there are other loaves left, plus plenty more at the store, and it's O. K. for her to eat all she wants.

She has yet to eat more than half a loaf at one sitting. She has also found that a poached egg on untoasted bread has a taste and texture that is very satisfying to her. Along with a glass of pineapple juice, this is often her breakfast and sometimes her supper. She no longer keeps a bare kitchen, but keeps it stocked with a good supply of foods, both for herself and friends. She has lost over twenty pounds since we first worked with her four months ago, and is now at a point where she doesn't care whether "I gain or lose a pound, because I just seem to stay around one hundred twenty-five, which is fine with me." Her overeating had been due primarily to eating around the bulk food that a person with a gut feeling of hunger often craves.

II. THROAT AND MOUTH HUNGER

Another common locale of hunger experience is in the upper throat and the back of the mouth. (Again: any individual can experience any or all of these hungers, depending on mood or psychological need).

The sensation may be a dull ache, a tight feeling or the impression that the area is hollow, but it is definitely confined to the area of the upper alimentary canal.

Foods that usually satisfy this site are sweet and cold: ice cream, milkshakes, chilled and iced soft drinks, fruit slushes, cream pies or puddings, ice-cold milk or beer, brandy Alexanders or stingers. People with cravings in this locale often eat their way through a whole meal — soup, salad, bread, meat, vegetables, and all — just to get to a cold, sweet dessert. Or they may fill up on cold, sweet beverages when they need it — in the afternoon, or before dinner. But then they eat a dinner, which is a wasted, unnecessary meal.

One workshop participant, having identified this as his kind of hunger, called us up one evening to report that he had had the most marvelous meal he could remember enjoying since he was a boy. He and his wife had to entertain a business associate and had gone to a fine restaurant. What he had ordered was a frozen daiquiri, two bowls of vichyssoise, and coconut cream pie a la mode. The waiter had demurred —

"Sir, we never serve cream pie a la mode" — but our friend had told him he was going to today, and he did.

Observing himself further; this man found that generally he preferred many foods cold, so he now eats hard-boiled rather than fried eggs; cold rather than hot roast beef; cold vegetables, cold fried chicken, and so on.

Instead of a coffee break, he goes to a nearby soda fountain and has a fruit slush or an ice cream soda. He has stopped eating the things he doesn't like, both at home and at business luncheons and dinners ("I often skip the whole entrée at these affairs") and is now within five pounds of what he considers a desirable weight.

III. GUM-AND-TEETH HUNGER

The third common hunger location is in the gum-and-teeth area. People with sensitivity in this area literally want to sink their teeth into something. Their hunger varies from a feeling of oral cavity emptiness to "itching" or to a dull aching akin to pain. They invariably need foods that require biting and chewing.

All the spaghetti or milkshakes in the world cannot provide satisfaction for this area. Sometimes this site is satisfied by "rabbit food," especially if used with a tangy or spicy dip. Crisp celery, carrots, and radishes may satisfy the need to bite, if such foods haven't been stigmatized since one's childhood by being labeled "healthful." Also high on the preferred list are pretzels, potato chips, French bread, nuts, spareribs, chewing gum, taffy, beef jerky, corn on the cob, steak, chicken wings, turkey drumsticks, and tart apples.

IV. TONGUE/ LIP HUNGER

Another common location of hunger is the tongue and/or lips. The old images of "smacking one's lips" and "licking one's chops" are quite literally true for this hunger. Both hunger and food anticipations are experienced in the lip and tongue area.

Foods most commonly craved are the ones that require licking and sucking, or foods that coat the tongue. Ice cream and soft candy can be favorites, but the foods that hum to this group need not be sweet. One person described the marvelous sensation of pulling an artichoke leaf through the teeth and, at the same time, along with the fibrous vegetable, feeling the smoothness of the mayonnaise it had been dipped in. Another woman got great pleasure from licking and sucking on a whole dill pickle; another enjoyed sucking on cheese or a banana; still another liked drinking through a straw (even beer and wine) rather than from a glass. Another found satisfaction for her hunger by not eating anything at all, but by simply licking barbecued potato chips and then discarding them, just to get that delicious, pungent, salty, spicy taste. Have you ever taken time to lick a potato chip?

LISTEN TO THE WISDOM OF YOUR BODY

Throughout this discussion we have referred to humming foods: foods that you really desire without analyzing nutritional value, calories, or other criteria.

Foods that hum to you are bound to be the ones that satisfy a particular hunger at a particular time. For instance, a person with a hunger sensation in the tongue would undoubtedly find that what hums is some food that can be licked or squished. Our bodies actually know what we need and transmit reliable signals. But we are rarely attuned to picking up these signals because we have been conditioned to ignore them and to deny their validity.

A small child being raised in a food-liberated household with no hang-ups about food can unerringly zero in on what hums to him. But most adults in our culture — especially if they are overweight — have been taught and forced to distrust themselves. "Don't give in to your cravings" is the battle cry of diet advocates. In other words, don't trust your body, ignore the signals you get, and shun your body's wisdom. Despite all this conditioning, the body signals are still there, but they may be garbled, and some help is needed so they can once again come through loud and clear.

In our work we have encountered literally thousands of people whose signals had gotten so garbled that they were not only ignored but misread. We have already mentioned some. There was also the man who ate dozens of barbequed spareribs mostly because he liked chewing on the bones; the woman who ate hamburgers because she craved the soft buns; the teen-age girl who consumed great quantities of ice cream cones after school every day only because she loved the crunchy sweet cones. She discovered this accidentally when a friend, as a special birthday treat, brought her a banana split; despite all that ice cream with the delicious sauces, nuts, and cherries, she felt unsatisfied because the cone was missing. She also discovered that her favorite ice cream parlor sells broken cones by the bag for next to nothing (as do many others). So now she often feasts on plain crunchy cones, lightly dipped in ice cream, rather than cones with ice cream in them.

A discussion of the basic problems and principles of food usage, and a fuller understanding of how you use food from a psychological perspective, does much to clear the way to liberated eating.

Not only is hunger felt in various locations of the body, but you may hunger for a definite and exact mood-satisfying food. A specific food can be craved because of psychological associations to various moods. In other words, certain foods carry certain psychological connotations. There are *reward foods* (chocolates, gooey cakes, sweets in general), *security foods* (breads, turkey with stuffing — things reminiscent of childhood), and *cultural-ethnic foods* (like pasta, chitterlings, chicken soup). Throughout the book we will be examining in detail the hunger for specific foods and your associations regarding them. Here we will outline them briefly.

REWARD FOODS

Almost everyone uses *reward foods* to reward or comfort himself. They tend to be chocolates, candies, cakes, pies, ice cream, and other sweets or dessert-type foods.

It's easy to see how the reward aspects of such foods become established. Children are taught to "finish your dinner (that healthy stuff) and then you can have your reward," namely the dessert (for eating what you often didn't like). It doesn't take long for the child to make the association "If I'm good, than I get the cookies or the cake."

As an adult, if you feel unrewarded, unappreciated, or overworked, it's easy to reward yourself with a sweet, gooey, creamy something.

Also, desserts are almost always forbidden to dieters because of the high calorie count. Nutritionists attack them because they constitute "empty calories." So it's easy to see why most people will choose dessert-type foods if they want to give themselves a real treat.

SECURITY FOODS

Security foods tend to be breads and rolls, fruit pies, turkey with stuffing, thick, hot soups, or biscuits — foods associated with Grandmother or Mother baking bread and savoring the aroma as it filled the house; with family dinners on Sundays, or perhaps every evening if dinner was the main meal, with everyone seated around the table.

When an adult feels uncertain or anxious, security foods often provide comfort. Unfortunately, the capacity of reward or security foods to do their psychological job is diminished if one views such eating as inappropriate or a sign of weakness or poor ego control. The desire for such foods springs from inner sources and needs recognition in the most direct and intense manner possible. When you deride yourself for yielding to such body needs, you often need five to ten times more of the rewarding or comforting food, because your pleasure is diluted by feelings of guilt, stupidity, anger, and self-hatred.

In other words, the use of security foods when one feels lonely, unloved, unappreciated, depressed, or otherwise insecure, is a valid use of foods.

CULTURAL-ETHNIC FOODS

Cultural-ethnic foods ("soul food") are a link to everyone's past. The range is almost infinite, from pasta to sauerkraut, brioche, lamb curry, chitterlings, bagels and lox, and cream cheese. Almost every diet urges you to reject your cultural heritage and ethnic identity by shunning such foods as if they were poison (most of them are high in calories). We believe, on the contrary, that such foods are essential for psychological functioning and happiness. We feel they need to be eaten whenever they hum, and enjoyed without the contaminating effects of the establishment nutritionists' warnings. This area of cultural foods will be discussed in detail in another chapter, but we want to say now that eating such foods is helpful when one feels alienated, isolated, lonely, or sad.

To summarize the very complex process called "hunger": There is an emotional trigger (or precipitant) for eating, such as boredom, anger, loneliness, tension, worry, etc. This is translated by the body into a need for a food, which often falls into a psychological category such as reward food, security food, or cultural-ethnic food. This is experienced by the person as a craving or hunger somewhere in the body, usually the alimentary canal: the stomach, the jaws, or the throat. Hunger is then satisfied by a food with certain qualities of taste, texture, or sensation.

5/ *A TIME TO EAT*

This chapter is for people who snack too much, the "nervous nibblers" — and those who use food as a substitute or replacement or solace for feelings such as fatigue, tension, or loneliness.

It may be practical, logical or convenient for social living to eat three meals a day at specified times. It may also be senseless, impractical, and damaging, because all too often this pattern simply does not fit your psychological or nutritional needs.

Since you were small you have probably been taught that breakfast, lunch, and dinner are the sanctioned times for eating, while eating between meals is wrong or bad. Everyday language reflects this attitude: Foods eaten at these established times constitute a meal; foods eaten at other times are snacks. If you take meat, bread, butter, and milk out of the refrigerator at noontime, you are preparing lunch, but if you get them out at midnight, you are raiding the refrigerator.

If you have been exposed to diet regimens and weight-reducing organizations, you may consider the meals you eat outside of established mealtimes illegitimate or forbidden. Why? All people do not get hungry at the same times or crave food at the same times any more than they all crave sex at the same times and under the same circumstances.

In recent decades, infants have luckily been freed from the regimentation of scheduled feedings. Most modern pediatricians feel that it is unreasonable to expect a baby's hunger to match the clock rather than his inner wants. Demand feeding — giving the child food when his body demands it rather than at a certain hour — is widely accepted and practiced. The mother who puts her infant on demand feeding shows that she trusts that small human being's body wisdom and body signals. Strangely, the same mother usually doesn't dare trust her own body wisdom.

Many pediatricians go further and say that there is also no need to achieve proper nutritional balance within every meal, or even within a given day or week. Dr. Margaret Ribble, author of *The Rights of Infants*, and one of the best-known of the doctors who take this approach, reported on studies that show that, given true food freedom, a child balances his own diet so that, over a period of time, he gets all components essential for healthy growth. The baby who wants nothing but applesauce for a while will suddenly delight in oatmeal or pureed meat or carrots.

These doctors feel that even if it takes a baby a long time to balance nutrition, healthy growth is not impeded. Rather, they contend, the child will grow up as a happy, unfussy, natural eater.

It has been our experience that much the same happens to adults if they can liberate themselves from imposed eating patterns and follow their own body signals. Here again the principle applies that freedom to eat also provides the freedom *not to eat*. Allowing yourself to eat exactly *what* you want, precisely *when* you feel like it, also means allowing yourself not to eat when you don't feel like it. You are no longer enslaved by clocks or "shoulds" or "should nots." If you don't feel hungry, skipping meals is a normal and natural event.

Picture it in your own mind: Do you feel guilty if you have had a big afternoon snack and then skip dinner? Do you feel so guilty that you still eat dinner, even if you don't really want it?

A great deal of overeating results not from people eating meals they want, but from their eating meals or foods they really don't want, but believe they *should* eat.

What do you consider the "right time" to eat? There is the common assumption that, once past infancy, people should be mature enough to be able to suppress and ignore body signals and schedule eating by the clock and other rituals. We believe that this has nothing to do with maturity. It is nothing but raw regimentation, and while there may be times and circumstances when a certain amount of regimentation is hard to avoid, it is certainly not desirable, and definitely not to be elevated to be a virtue.

Unless there are other compelling reasons, the right time to eat is when you feel like eating. The wrong time to eat is when you don't feel like eating.

For some people, the right time may be once a day, and for others five or six times. For many people, there is great variation. Some days they will feel like eating frequently, other days hardly at all. (How many times have you heard someone say, "I just don't feel like eating today," only to go on and eat anyway?)

Take a look at the natural "thinnies" you know. In all probability, many of them have no set eating pattern at all. They eat at vastly different hours and in vastly different amounts, depending on such factors as whether they feel happy or frustrated, tired, anguished, energetic, festive, well-rested, lazy, or pressured. It may be so natural to them that they are not consciously aware of it at all, but they are following their body signals.

Many nutritional theories exist about the times when food intake is most beneficial to the body and its proper maintenance. We do not intend to take issue with their validity for a great many people. However, if these recommended patterns run counter to a person's psychological needs, the damage they do outweighs the good they do.

Many of these food theories deal with the importance of breakfast. In Holland the customary breakfast includes several kinds of bread, butter, boiled or smoked ham and other cold meats, cheeses, and often eggs — a dream meal for those who preach the importance of protein in the morning.

But in France, by marked contrast, the customary breakfast consists of coffee with milk, a hard roll or croissant or two, butter, and maybe a spoonful of jam — a nightmare of a meal for the protein-at-breakfast proponents. Yet, in both countries people lead active lives, both countries boast great achievements, and the average life expectancy of Frenchmen and Dutchmen is almost identical.

Many obese people are afraid that they would eat not only too much, but none of the "healthy" foods, if they removed all restrictions. Taking supplemental vitamins can alleviate many of these fears,* but as we have already mentioned in several short case histories, people often find that they really like many "healthy" or "diet-type" foods once the stigma of being restricted to diet foods is removed. (Remember the German engineer who now loves to eat radishes with his liverwurst, though he used to detest anything that came under the heading of rabbit food?)

At the Institute, we have seen many avowed sweets eaters who, after a few weeks of free eating, developed not only a liking but an actual craving for meat, or legumes, or fruit, or dairy foods, or vegetables.

THE CASE OF MAVIS

One example was Mavis, an ample-bosomed woman of forty-five, who was raising two foster children along with her own four, and in addition kept busy with PTA work and volunteer work for political candidates.

Mavis snacked on pastries throughout the day, but always conscientiously ate well-balanced meals with the family "to set a good example for the children." Some of the food she ate at these meals she liked, though she didn't really desire it. Some she detested, including most vegetables, "because

---

*We suggest one of the multi-vitamin capsules that contain the nutrients generally recognized as necessary to meet daily requirements.

someone was always telling me I should have more of that because it's good for me and won't make me fat."

In the course of a workshop and sessions of an ongoing group, Mavis tuned in to the idea of food that hums and eating only what and when you feel like it. She also decided to assert her right to her own body. Her one worry was that she might damage her health, but she decided vitamin supplements would probably keep her in reasonable health.

For a while she ate more pastry than anything else, openly and without making excuses. After a week, though, she was amazed to find that one morning, rather than wanting a butter horn, what hummed to her was shrimp.

More startling, when she opened a can of shrimp and started to eat it, things weren't quite right. What she really wanted was shrimp on lettuce. Lettuce? "I couldn't believe this was me," Mavis reported at our next meeting.

Two more weeks went by, during which she ate shrimp and tuna salad at breakfast and a lot of pastry later in the day. Then she was almost embarrassed to report a new development: She had developed a craving for broccoli and was eating it in large quantity, both cooked and raw.

She laughed at the very idea of herself going to the refrigerator at 10:00 P.M. and getting out a stalk of broccoli to munch on while she fixed the children's school lunches for the next day.

As of this writing, almost a year has passed since Mavis's broccoli phase. By traditional standards, her present eating pattern would be called erratic — she always eats a substantial though unconventional breakfast, no lunch, but several snacks throughout the day, sometimes dinner and sometimes not, often a late snack but sometimes not. She goes through phases of eating a lot of one particular food (most recently, hard-cooked eggs with mustard) and she feels good about her eating and her body.

Food management, meal schedules, and convenience in food preparation are important realities for any housewife. With six children of various ages and the necessity for keeping the household operating smoothly, Mavis had to maintain law and order in the kitchen. Since she was a busy person who thrived on having routines run smoothly, Mavis retained the three-meals-a-day pattern for her children. However, she relaxed a number of eating rules. For example, the children were allowed to participate in making up the grocery shopping list, and could express their preferences for main dishes before they were prepared. New family rules were negotiated regarding which snack food could be eaten, and when and where. (We'll discuss family unity and food management in greater detail in Chapter 10.)

We felt that one of the most important changes for Mavis was that she was able to stop feeling guilty about eating at unusual times.

ANNETTE'S STORY

Another dieter, Annette, in her mid-forties and living in a tree-shaded suburb in California, had a related problem that might help some readers get in touch with their own situation.

(Each person with an eating problem faces a unique situation. People have to get in touch with themselves, tune in to their own needs and focus their attention on their own body signals to achieve such a change and form a new, free relationship to food and eating. Our method is designed to point people in the right direction and help clarify both the problem of overeaters and the alternatives open to them. Our sample case histories, therefore, are not intended to give an approach pattern to be followed exactly, but we have found that a candid view of another person's situation helps people to reexamine and rethink their own situation.)

Annette's husband, an energetic self-made man with a thriving real-estate firm of his own, belonged to many organizations and liked to entertain a great deal at home, both for business reasons and because it suited his outgoing personality.

Don didn't want Annette to work, yet after their two sons left for college, she felt bored and ended up doing four hours of volunteer work with indigent elderly patients at a hospital twelve miles from home every day.

She loved this work, but felt emotionally spent at the end of each shift. She started to stop at a coffee shop near the hospital for a cup of coffee and a snack, but the snack soon became supper-sized, because she really craved food at this time.

A few times Annette tried not to eat dinner at home and told Don that she had already eaten. He was annoyed and hurt. He told her he couldn't enjoy food by himself; certainly, guests would be offended if the hostess didn't eat herself; they themselves wouldn't be invited to people's houses if she didn't eat dinner — in short, it would ruin their pleasant life-style.

Annette is an agreeable, soft-spoken woman who abhors conflict. Like an obedient child, she ate her dinners at home or at the home of friends, and she tried to cut down on her mid-afternoon meals.

It didn't work. The harder she tried, the more she craved food when she left the hospital, and the more she ended up eating at the coffee shop.

As might be expected, her weight started going up. She had never been slender, but also never fat, carrying 120 pounds on a five-foot, four-inch frame. When her weight reached 135, she started to worry; when it reached 145, Don hit the ceiling. He had always ridiculed fat women, and he told her that even though he loved her, he couldn't stand the idea of her getting fat.

Their whole relationship became strained, and their sex life became all but nonexistent. Don would bring home diet plans and magazine articles for Annette; she went to two local doctors who specialized in obesity problems; she joined a weight-reducing organization — all to no avail. She would lose a few pounds and put them right back on again, plus a few more. Much as she tried, she could not stop her mid-afternoon meals, though she lied to Don that she had cut them back to a cup of coffee and maybe a little salad.

When Annette came to us, she weighed 160 pounds and was a thoroughly unhappy woman: "At forty-six, I'm a fat old lady, all washed up. My husband won't touch me, and when I look in the mirror I start to cry."

One solution might have been for Annette to stop working at the hospital, but her pride wouldn't allow that. "Then I would *really* be useless," was her response.

She also rejected the idea of a third person trying to deal with Don and convince him that his wife's need for a big meal in mid-afternoon was legitimate — that he should stop insisting on her eating again at dinnertime.

However, when she herself started to look upon her afternoon eating as fulfillment of a valid emotional need, rather than a shameful, uncontrolled weakness, and when she tuned into the idea of humming, things did change. Rather than hurry to the coffee shop and quickly order a lot of food, she would try to tune into what precisely was humming to her before she even left the hospital and then order precisely that food. It turned out to be soft-textured, warm food, and sweets. So, rather than a full dinner, she often had soup and pie, or a bowl of mashed potatoes with gravy and a pudding, or an omelette and ice cream.

She found that by dinnertime, which was late in the evening, she again had an appetite, but very different things hummed to her then — mostly highly seasoned meats and fish. This, of course, presented no problem with Don. To see her skip starchy foods and desserts pleased him — even after she told him it was not because she was dieting.

After she had lost about sixteen pounds, she took the plunge and told him the whole truth — that she was still having her reward foods in the afternoon, but then, and also at dinner and at all other times, she was eating exactly what she wanted and nothing else.

It was a hard idea for Don to accept, because it ran contrary to the usual deprivation approaches. But the honesty that had returned to their relationship, plus the fact that Annette was losing weight, impressed him. Gradually, their entire relationship improved.

STRESS-RELATED EATING PROBLEMS

Many people's food needs are related to a job or other activity involving stress. The right time to eat, for them, is whenever there is a strong food craving — such as just before work or during a coffee break or right after work. To try to deny your need at such a time is psychologically unsound. If your own overeating falls into this pattern, focus on it.

Do you consider the coffee-break doughnuts, the after-work snacks, or the on-the-way-to-work eating to be your worst overeating? How about breakfast, lunch, and dinner? Do you eat foods then that you don't really desire, that don't hum to you, but that you eat out of habit and "because they are there"? How about calling *that* overeating? In our view, it is!

Joan came to our workshop after many unsuccessful diet attempts. She was fifty-seven, a highly regarded accountant in a large concern. When the firm switched to computers, Joan's job was eliminated. She was kept on, at the same pay, but in a totally boring, mechanical job.

At her age she did not think that she could find another interesting position. She had been with the company for twenty-two years and had substantial, non-transferable retirement benefits coming. So she made up her mind to grin and bear it for the eight years to retirement.

She did manage to put up with the job, but she started gaining weight, slowly but steadily. The reason was fairly clear: Every morning, on her way to work, she ate a large chocolate candy bar. She was, quite plainly, rewarding and comforting herself *in advance* for having to go through eight hours of drudgery.

She had been fighting this pattern valiantly when she finally came to us for help. The more she tried to stop herself from doing this "ridiculous, childish, undisciplined thing," the more obsessive it became. On days when she did force herself to get to the office without a bite of chocolate, she would sneak off to the ladies' room after a short while and gobble down two or three candy bars then, and more later.

Quite probably, Joan could have solved her eating and weight problem by quitting her job. But she did not feel that this was an acceptable option.

We were able to help her see that her rewarding herself with chocolate was a perfectly legitimate activity, not in the least bit ridiculous, childish, or undisciplined. We encouraged her to buy chocolate by the boxful, to carry a good supply, even to keep a box in her desk. We also encouraged her to eat it openly, not to sneak it as she had done in the past.

At first, she found this hard to do, but eventually she managed. When someone asked her now and then, "What, *you* eating chocolate?" she answered, "Sure, haven't you heard of the Chocolate Diet? The latest thing — works like a charm."

In some ways, it did work like a charm. Having accepted as legitimate her own way of dealing with stress, or an unpleasant situation, and having overcome the feeling that she should hide this from other people, she no longer was obsessed with the idea of gobbling more and more chocolate bars. She ate less chocolate, fewer meals, and lost her excess weight.

WHEN NOT TO EAT

So far, we have dealt with examples of eating unusual things at unusual times and have tried to point out that you have a right and need to eat in that way if those foods hum to you at those times. But some overweight people do eat when they shouldn't. We are talking about times when a person uses eating as a substitute activity for something else — a nap, a shower, a walk, sex, a time of absolute quiet, to name a few.

To use food to alleviate these needs is not the world's worst idea if you cannot meet your true need more directly, but it is highly inefficient. If you feel exhausted and sweaty, no amount of cake, or nuts, or candy, or potato chips can give you the same lift that a bath and brief rest can. After a day of sitting at a desk, if you feel cramped, headachy, and irritated, no ice cream or pretzels or hors d'oeuvres can restore your body to the same feeling of well-being that a brisk walk would.

Focus on this for a moment. Do you eat at such times? And if you do, is it really, truly impossible for you to meet that need more directly? If food is the only alternative, can you select the food that comforts you the most?

We frequently encounter people who want to change but are not aware of the choices open to them.

Instead, they focus on negatives — what not to do or what not to eat. Other alternatives are unexplored because the person doesn't realize options exist. And of course it is difficult to develop new psychological insights, and then to break out of accustomed life patterns.

When people find out that they use food to satisfy non-food-related body needs, such as a need for sleep, their first reaction tends to be one of hopelessness. Circumstances, they feel, are against them. They are trapped by forces beyond their control.

You may have the same reaction at this point. If you're the mother of small children, you might say, "Sure, I often eat when I feel rushed, tied down, harried, tired, and ugly. But how could I go to the beauty parlor, or take a nap or a bath in the middle of the day, or go for a walk by myself? It's impossible!"

Career people have much the same attitude, frequently citing lack of time as the reason for not efficiently meeting an existing and acknowledged body need.

We fully realize that change is rarely easy. If it were that simple, there wouldn't be sixty million overweight Americans.

We encourage our workshop participants (and would like to suggest to you) to do simply this: Focus on your needs; allow yourself to become conscious of what you really need or crave, what would give you optimal satisfaction. Have you let yourself think in terms of "What is it I really want?" Most people don't, because they feel it's impossible or too selfish. And if you are in touch with your real need, do you feel you're entitled to meet it directly?

Overweight people tend to suppress their real body needs, because it would be "slothful" to nap during the daytime; it would be "self-indulgent" to take a bubble bath in the afternoon; it would be "selfish to think of myself first."

Have you felt that way about your wants?

Realizing what the true bodily need is — and feeling entitled to meet it — sometimes leads to a solution. A walk or shower or afternoon sex or quiet periods of time were "impossible" only when they were viewed as immoral or a sign of weak character, not for what they actually are: a genuine, valid need. Thin people can respond to such needs, accept them, and satisfy them.

Here are some people we have worked with who found alternate ways of satisfying their needs once they became aware of them and accepted those needs as valid.

ADRIANNE COULDN'T "WASTE" FOOD

Adrianne, a pretty blond housewife from New England now living in Sacramento, had been athletic in her teens and early twenties and had always had a trim figure.

She married Bob, an architecture student, when she was twenty-four, and had her first baby when she was twenty-six. A second child was born fifteen months later, and number three barely two years after that.

Both Bob and Adrianne were happy with their lifestyle; they wanted children and fully enjoyed them.

"My only problem is my weight," Adrianne declared when we first met. "Everything else is fine. But since I stay home with the kids and don't get into athletics anymore, everything I eat turns to fat. I just keep gaining and gaining."

She was then thirty-three and weighed 147 pounds — thirty more than at the time of her marriage. "And I am still gaining! Not much really, just a half a pound or so every month. It just sneaks up on me."

In the weekly ongoing group that Adrianne joined after attending our basic workshop, we further explored her eating patterns.

She was not a frequent snack eater, but two things stood out: She had slipped into a pattern of having a bottle of beer with her lunch and one or two more during the afternoon. She didn't like hard liquor, she said, but "I get so tense, and get short-tempered that I snap and shout at the kids. I just can't hold onto my temper anymore, and the beer calms me down. I guess it's my pacifier."

She also admitted to always "cleaning up" the children's plates.

Bob, now out of school, was still on a fairly low salary, and the family budget was tight. "Waste just bothers me" is the way Adrianne put it. If one of the children left half his French toast at breakfast, she finished it. "A lot of my eating is nervous eating, too. I don't even realize that I've eaten something until I'm finished."

If at lunchtime part of a sandwich and some Jell-O were left, Adrianne ate that. Ditto with meatloaf or mashed potatoes, or cupcakes with only the frosting eaten off, half-drunk glasses of milk, and so on. This "economical" procedure made Adrianne feel like a vacuum cleaner, which is common with women who stay home.

Adrianne had readily understood and accepted the idea of food that hums, and admitted that leftovers definitely did not hum. "Hum? They don't even beckon! It's just become a habit, I guess, and we really cannot afford to waste all that food."

We did point out to her that there was a fallacy there.

"When I was a little boy," Leo, another member of the group, told her, "I was constantly being urged to finish my plate because I should think of the starving children in China.

"One day it finally dawned on me that there was something wrong with this argument. If I ate my food, well, then certainly that food couldn't go to the children of China. And if I didn't eat it and it went to the dog or into the garbage can, that, too, didn't reach those starving children. In other words, eating or not eating my dinner wasn't going to make any difference to those children one way or another."

By the same token, Adrianne conceded that her family budget wasn't going to benefit by her eating up the leftovers. The food had been bought and prepared, and whether part of it was thrown out or eaten by her was neither going to cost nor save any money. Further, she had spent a small fortune on weight specialists and pills. She had lost thirty pounds five times and regained them each time, and felt discouraged and hopeless.

Adrianne decided she would stop eating leftovers, but she found that hard going. "I guess I really want them, after all. I think I get some sort of psychological hunger when I see them, and eating somehow eases my irritation and nervousness."

What irritation? What nervousness? It took Adrianne quite a while to find out what was going on. She finally got in touch with a sentiment that she had resolutely suppressed. As much as she loved her children, she did resent them at times because they kept her tied to the house and deprived her of a chance to enjoy her beloved sports.

"So go play tennis or go hiking or swimming at least a couple of times a week," another member of the group suggested.

"I'd love to," said Adrianne, "but I can't. It's impossible."

The reasons she gave were that she had too much work and that she couldn't afford a babysitter.

We urged her to consider the importance of all the factors involved: her duties, her overeating, her overweight, her dissatisfaction, her beer-drinking (of which she was ashamed, and which had become quite an issue between her and Bob).

Basic to the whole question was: Could she accept that she really did deserve to allocate time for herself? *Housewives often put themselves last in line. Eventually they view as worthwhile and valid only those activities that serve their families.*

Bob was supportive and assured Adrianne that he considered it proper and right for her to trade babysitting with a neighbor and to hire a babysitter at least a few hours a week so she could have some time for herself.

Adrianne could accept that she had been spending more money on beer, diet pills, and dietetic foods than she would on a babysitter, but she still had a hang-up: "It doesn't seem right to spend money just to please myself."

In time, this attitude did change, and Adrianne was able to think of herself as "me, sports-loving Adrianne" rather than "Adrianne, wife of Bob" and "Adrianne, mother of Jimmy,

Eric, and Jennifer." She then was able to allow herself some private time and to enjoy it without feelings of guilt.

Changing one aspect of her living pattern was an answer for this particular woman; for other "nervous nibblers" the solution might be totally different.

JACKIE, THE CHOCOLATE FREAK

Jackie is a stewardess flying international flights out of New York. She is twenty-six, five foot six, 121 pounds. She wears her auburn hair in a short cut and puts on just enough eye make-up to emphasize the soft green of her eyes. She makes no attempt to hide the few freckles on her face.

One of the workshop members muttered as she came into the room, "What the hell is *she* doing *here?*"

Jackie is slender, well-groomed, pretty, sexy, and poised. She is also a chocolate freak who lived in constant terror that someday she might get fat.

Jackie had no weight problem (she has never weighed more than 124 pounds), but she had a serious eating problem, one that preoccupied her most of her waking hours.

When people were outlining their problems, Jackie said, "I'm a super-chocoholic." And to prove it, she produced a small leather-bound notebook, her international guide to chocolate. She makes notations in it wherever she goes. "You want to know where you get the best chocolate creams in London?" she asked. "Here it is. The only really superb chocolate layer cake in Brisbane? Here's the address. Here's a place on the outskirts of Athens that has a beautiful chocolate bar with almonds and honey. And here is one in downtown Munich that has the greatest soft chocolate nougat by the pound."

Despite her expertise in the world of chocolate, Jackie got little pleasure from eating chocolate. What she began to realize during the food-awareness training sessions on Saturday was the fact that she hardly ever tasted the chocolate. She went on her chocolate-eating binges when she felt tense or nervous and under stress.

And, like many other nervous nibblers, Jackie's taste at these times was numbed. She ate a lot, but tasted little.

Jackie realized that many occasions make her nervous. A few she singled out were when she knows there is going to be a VIP on board; before a date; when she is going to be flying with a captain she doesn't know; when there are many children on a flight; when she thinks there may be a check hostess on her next flight; and when her parents come to New York!

She came to see that her chocolate-eating did have emotional value for her, but she also became aware that it wasn't a very efficient way of meeting her need.

A small glass of certain liqueurs — Vandermint or creme de cacao — turned out to be far more effective for her. It has the soothing sweetness of chocolate but requires no chewing. Most important, a small glass of liqueur really helps her to relax. At times when she can't drink liqueur, such as shortly before or during a flight, she now uses hot chocolate with gooey melted marshmallows, which she finds soothing and relaxing.

You may wonder why we didn't get to the root of Jackie's feelings of anxiety and tension. Our assumption, based on modern humanistic psychology, is that tension is a legitimate response to certain situations and does not have to be removed or treated through psychotherapy. Rather, such tension is a valid feeling and the issue is how to soothe or satisfy that state.

For Jackie, keeping a small bottle of liqueur and a few envelopes of instant hot-chocolate mix in her handbag has proven more helpful and tension-reducing than chewing her way through a pound of chocolates.

If you consider yourself a nervous nibbler, check it out. Maybe some unmet need has to be allowed to surface (as it did in Adrianne's case). On the other hand, the response to your nervous nibbling may indeed be eating. But the issue is how to be most efficient about it, how to obtain the exact comforting sensation from food (as in Jackie's case).

Mothers of young children seem particularly prone to tension eating. Often this kind of eating is indiscriminate; at other times, it's very specific, perhaps concentrating on sweets or nuts.

This kind of eating is rarely satisfying, but it is often the only way people allow treats or pleasures into their lives. Food represents a small burst of sensation, a giving-to-oneself in a life otherwise filled with meeting the needs of others.

EMILY COULDN'T BE "SELFISH"

Emily, in her late thirties, almost ninety pounds overweight, the wife of a minister, and the mother of four children, found herself frightened by the idea of planning part of her life to allow her to pleasure herself with food.

"That's selfish!" she objected. "If I start to do something like that, where could it all lead? I might become a totally self-centered and selfish person."

She admitted that most of her eating was done either on the run or at times when she wasn't hungry. Her schedule was structured according to others' needs, not her own.

Her way of using food was inefficient and psychologically wasteful. Eating on the run and nibbling forbidden sweets were her clandestine contacts with an intimate, lovable enemy.

Is most of your life spent with tasks and activities that are humming to you? Or is it mostly filled with obligations and things that, at best, beckon? The way you eat is often tied very closely to your philosophy of existence and how you live. Many people who gain freedom in their relationship to food find that this carries over and allows them to exercise many more options in other areas of their lives.

For example, Louise, a divorced and lively school teacher in her early forties, wanted help with her forty-pound weight problem, which she had battled unsuccessfully for years.

She discovered that she was seriously out of tune with herself, not only in her eating (she was at first totally unsure about what and when she enjoyed eating), but in many other areas of her life.

She was accommodating, helpful, and reliable. "I'm always the good kid," she said. This went to the point that at school she allowed herself to be burdened with extra teaching assignments which she genuinely disliked. She also hated to hurt a man's feelings by refusing to go out with him, so she sometimes wasted whole evenings with people who bored her, rather than hurt someone's feelings. And, of course, much of her eating was to reward or fortify herself for more sacrifice or self-denial.

For Louise, tuning into the idea of freedom to eat and freedom to not eat also carried with it freedom to say "no" to others and to live life more precisely according to her inner needs.

Self-denial (as with Louise or Adrianne) is high on the list of reasons for "replacement eating." So is loneliness.

We want to reemphasize that we do not expect any-one's problem to be identical to any of those we describe. But we believe that some of these situations may evoke feelings of similarity in many and thereby lead to new awareness and deeper insights into personal ways of relating to food.

EATING TO BEAT LONELINESS

Duane was a person who ate largely out of loneliness. He also had a hard time expressing angry feelings. When he felt anger, he literally swallowed it and then swallowed food on top of it, as if to make sure that it stayed buried.

A draftsman, Duane had been raised in a small town in Iowa. He was thirty-four when he sought private consultations with us because he felt "too ashamed to discuss such personal matters in a group."

He weighed 244 pounds — seventy-four pounds more than his doctor thought healthy. He had been dieting ever since he was a teenager, and by the time he came to us he had been living on grapefruit, cottage cheese, lean hamburger patties, and coffee for more than four years. At least, that's what he ate for most meals.

He talked at length of his Spartan diet, adding, "Of course, when I take a date out, we go to the best restaurants and I eat a normal dinner then, so I won't make her feel uncomfortable."

Hardly the road to obesity. Only it turned out that late at night, after taking his date home, he often made the rounds of pizza parlors or hamburger stands, eating large amounts of food and washing it down liberally with chocolate-caramel milkshakes.

Duane had had a few affairs, but felt shy and insecure with women. He began to see that his eating was a response to the inner emptiness he felt because of the lack of close relationships.

On evenings when he had no date, his feelings were almost overwhelming; loneliness overshadowed everything else. This loneliness, he found, could be partly assuaged by sweet, gooey reward foods. These were the evenings when the milkshakes outnumbered the pizza and hamburgers.

But no matter what kind of evening he had had, he always begrudged himself every bite and every sip, focusing on the calories he was consuming and feeling stupid and undisciplined. He had once gone to a "fat doctor," who told him that his was a typical example of "nocturnal hyperphagia." That gave him a scientific label, but it did not do a thing to change either his eating or his feelings about it.

After several months of counseling, Duane came to realize and accept that food and eating were his means of dealing with tension. When there were difficulties at work or in his social life, he didn't shout at anybody, he didn't get drunk, he didn't take it out on the office boy — he made a trip to the hamburger stand. But now that he feels free to eat his reward and comfort foods, he needs less of them and enjoys them, thus getting full psychological value from what he eats.

Duane is not surrendering to food; he has legitimized his need for foods, foods that hum to him under very specific circumstances.

If he has a meal late at night, he usually does not feel hungry in the morning and most of the next day, not because he wants to make up for his excesses of the previous night, but because he is quite genuinely still full and aware of it.

Prior to working with us, Duane (whose weight, incidentally, fluctuates currently between 200 and 205 pounds — a forty-pound loss) had always been convinced that if he let himself go, he would eat all the time, "day and night, seven days a week."

Many people who come to us have this same fear. In the few instances where people did gain, they were using our method as an excuse to surrender to food, to throw in the sponge rather than to tune in to precise signals.

People who are able to explore themselves and get in touch with their needs often report that they experience a tremendous feeling of relief even before any weight loss occurs. It's good to know where you stand in relation to food, and to make friends with an old, torturing enemy.

6/ *THE PLEASURABLE USE OF LIQUIDS*

This chapter examines how to handle beverages — including alcohol — as vital life substances. It is especially for those who think they could lose weight if only they were able to cut out or reduce drinking, and those who resent all dieting because this usually means no more drinking — whether it's wine or soda pop.

People who have difficulty with eating often have similar problems with drinking and with tuning in to what they want to drink, and when, and how. *The same guilt that filters out pleasures in eating often occurs with drinking.*

Many people feel they over drink and wish they could cut down on Cokes, or milkshakes, or alcohol. This is particularly frequent with alcohol: People assert that they would lose weight if they could only give up their beer, or their martini-stop at the bar near the office, or their dinner wine, or their liqueurs and after-dinner brandies.

In the context of this book we will not deal with the problem of alcoholism, though the fear of becoming an alcoholic would certainly interfere with allowing yourself the freedom to enjoy drinking. People who are afraid they may become alcoholic "if I let myself go" are often reflecting feelings of guilt about drinking, rather than commenting on what could actually happen to them. We consider people to be "social drinkers" if they function reasonably successfully in their personal and professional life and in their social relations. *We have yet to see a single person become alcoholic because of allowing himself or herself more freedom and pleasuring in drinking.* However, we have certainly seen how being *afraid* of becoming an alcoholic automatically puts you on a liquor diet. There is then much the same battle that can occur with food: guilt, deprivation, warfare, binging (which can lead to alcoholism), restrictions, rebellion — all of which keep you out of touch with what you really want and enjoy.

Others are not concerned about becoming alcoholic, but believe that the calories in alcohol are chiefly responsible for their weight problem. This is especially true if you are worried about getting proper nutrition while you are on a diet; then the alcohol represents excess calories that are responsible for breaking the diet.

Dieters also often find that when they drink they lose control of their appetites. Less frequently, they may even lose interest in eating. Most frequently, a person thinks that drinking makes him "relax too much, and then I lose control over how much I eat and what I eat." We have found that in these instances alcohol becomes an excuse for *allowing* yourself what the diet is *forbidding* you. When you stop the dieting approach — when food deprivation and self-control are no longer issues — then overeating because of alcohol-induced relaxation ceases to be a problem. We have discussed how food is often used to alleviate body needs other than hunger; how people eat instead of taking a nap, or a walk, or a bubble bath. The same thing happens frequently with beverages. People have a cup of coffee to "stay awake," tea to "get a quick pick-me-up," a cocktail because "I'm all bushed."

This is a legitimate way of using beverages, But it may not be the most efficient thing to satisfy your need. As with eating, allowing yourself to have a nap, a shower, or a walk is best in the sense that it does the most for you. You might then have the beverage afterward — if it hums to you — or for the sheer pleasure of it.

There is no question that alcohol can help you to relax. We believe this is a *very* important function of alcohol. It's much more efficient than food for relaxation. And it has been used that way for a long time. The use of fermented drink has been recorded since antiquity.

In other ways, beverages are unique, especially alcohol. Beverages can enhance a mood. For example, we worked with one woman who found that her super-unwinder at the end of a hectic work day was sipping a sweet vermouth over ice while soaking in a bubble bath.

To some, beverages — including alcohol — may be more emotionally important than food. This doesn't mean you're a potential alcoholic! It means that, for you, beverages are essential and basic.

In a biological sense, fluids are the most vital substance for sustaining life. You can live without food for a much longer period of time than you can without fluids. Even when fasting, a person needs fluids to survive.

We have found that on some occasions people eat instead of drinking. If anything, the total pleasures of drinking are not given enough emphasis.

In drinking anything, whether alcoholic or a soft drink, examine and experiment to determine your exact preferences. Don't be regulated by convention.

Most people allow their drinking to be largely, if not entirely, regulated by custom and convention. For example, there is no reason to drink beverages at the temperature considered proper.

How would you feel about a gin and tonic *with* dinner? What about an after-dinner martini? Or Grand Marnier at cocktail time? Or beer with dessert? Or sweet sherry with dinner?

How do you know what hums to you in what one of our workshop participants called "the wonderful world of booze?" First of all, it is helpful to try to ignore such labels as "martini time," "time for the wine," and "time for after-dinner drinks." Instead, ask yourself, "What would I really like, *right now?*"

If nothing comes to mind very clearly, it could be that you actually don't want anything. The idea of having a drink might have emerged only because someone else suggested it. Obviously, liquor can be enjoyed any time, but we're talking about the inner-based hum, not the social beckoning.

If several things seem to hum, try the approach of asking yourself, "Would I feel cheated if I did not have this now?"

AFTER-DINNER DRINKS BEFORE DINNER?

Ruth, a thirty-two-year-old newspaper reporter, reported in one of our ongoing groups how this worked out for her. Ruth was going through a phase of treating herself on frequent occasions with B&B, the blend of brandy and Benedictine. But when she was invited to a formal social event, she felt embarrassed to ask for a B&B before dinner.

Instead, she said, "I'd really like something sort of sweet." The host suggested, "How about a Mai-Tai or a dai-quiri or Kir — that's very good, it's creme de cassis with Cha-blis."

All these drinks sounded fine, and Ruth settled on the Mai-Tai.

After a few sips, she felt somehow cheated and dissatis-fied. She asked herself whether she would have felt cheated without that Mai-Tai. She would not have. The same was true of the daiquiri and the Kir. But she felt convinced that she *did* feel cheated without the B&B. So she went back, told the host that the Mai-Tai didn't quite hit the spot, and asked for a B&B.

Since, as we have said, over drinking — whether alco-holic or non-alcoholic — is psychologically similar to the over-eating process, here is the approach we recommend: Pleasure yourself with liquids; explore beverages; explore the way you use them and the satisfactions they give you; get in touch with situations that trigger over drinking; attempt to find the beverage and mode of drinking that will most efficiently meet your need; determine specifically what drinks hum to you, when, in what situations, and at what times. And don't let conventions dictate what to do, with drink any more than with food.

As a starting point on the road to becoming a liberated drinker, we recommend several drinking exercises (See Chap-ter 13).

7/ *A PLACE TO EAT*

This chapter deals with "sneak eaters" and explores the problems of unremembered "amnesia eating." You'll also find suggestions for those who must (or choose to) eat alone. And we reveal a technique to help you stop eating before you feel stuffed.

> The suspect gave her name as Donna White, 39, of 2340 Poplar Street. She has medium brown hair, gray eyes, is 5' 4", and weighs 208 pounds. The floor of her automobile, a copper-toned 1971 Pinto, was littered with a chewy chocolate candy allegedly known as "turtles." It is apparent that this woman's eating candy while operating a vehicle was the sole cause of a seven-car collision. She is being held without bail . . .

This police report was never written. But countless overweight people live in constant fear that it might be written — about them. The fact that they like to eat in such "outlandish" places as their automobile adds to their negative feelings about themselves and supports their conviction that "the other people" — the thinnies — look upon them with disgust or out-and-out condemnation.

They are convinced that in a situation such as a traffic accident or at the scene of a crime, an obese person found eating would almost automatically be the prime suspect.

WHERE DO YOU EAT?

Our society sanctions only certain times and places for eating, just as there are sanctioned times and places for sex, for sleeping, etc. The places that are considered proper for eating are mainly the breakfast table, the lunch counter, and the dinner table, plus a few special-occasion places, such as picnic sites, restaurants, and parties.

People with an eating problem usually stick to these prescribed places while they live under the self-imprisoned conditions of dieting. But when they break out of jail and allow themselves the pleasure of food, they can't be bothered with finding a proper place to eat. In fact, very often these proper places are unsuitable because it is important to overeaters that their spouse, or parents, or children, or lover, or friends, or even total strangers, not see them eating. Also, they have to be able to hide evidence of having sinned by eating.

Consequently, overweight people often sneak food in refuges, like the car, elevator, bathroom, movie house, second landing on the stairway, basement, garage, fire escape, bus, and bed.

Candy eaten in the car is no more fattening than candy nibbled at the bridge table. But if you feel like an undercover agent in enemy country, you have to conceal your eating and be wary of leaving tracks, such as candy wrappers.

Strong prejudice exists against overweight people who eat in public view. In part, these prejudices result from the same ideas of regimentation we discussed in the context of "proper" eating times. Then, there is the general prejudice against obesity, which makes almost anything the overweight person does suspect, simply because he does it.

The difficulty with "espionage eating" is not the odd locale, but the interference with pleasurable, languid, sensuous eating. There isn't adequate time to extract the full flavor and delight available in foods of all kinds. It becomes necessary to consume much more to obtain the essence of candy, nuts, or cheese if you have to be alert for the cop while you're eating.

By way of contrast, stop to consider this picture in your mind's eye: Another person at your office, a genuine "thinny," is walking down the hallway, pulls a candy bar out of his pocket, and starts to munch on it. Would you consider him undisciplined? Would you think, "There he goes again, that slob?" Do you think others would have that reaction? In all likelihood, the answer to all these questions is "no."

Now picture yourself — if you have a weight problem — doing the same thing and then ask the same questions. In all likelihood, the answer to all three questions is "yes."

What is the difference? Prejudice, mostly. But there may be one other basic difference. Chances are that the thin fellow gets out that candy bar because he feels like eating candy. He may never have heard the term, but candy is humming to him at that precise time and in that precise place. That is why he eats it right there in the hallway.

You might eat it for the same reason, and that's fine. You might also eat it there because fewer people will see you eating candy; because eating while walking along seems less like "real eating"; because the calories might be offset partially by the exercise of walking; or because eating while you are doing something else makes you hurry through the eating and get it over with.

(Note that we are talking of eating as escape or protection. There are other reasons, which we will deal with shortly.)

At any rate, all these reasons are valid and make sense, given the need to eat secretly.

There is also a close analogy to eating instead of satisfying a different type of body need, such as taking a nap, which we discussed earlier. Those are legitimate times to eat if you cannot meet your bodily or psychological needs more directly and efficiently. The hallway — or any of the other places you might choose — are legitimate places to eat if you cannot meet your need more directly.

In other words, if you are hungering for candy while sitting at your desk, the optimal solution is to eat it right there, not defiantly, but out of the conviction that you are entitled to pleasure yourself with food and that you have a right to make decisions about your own body, including its food intake. But if that is not possible for you, if the knowledge of being watched and the likelihood of being teased or admonished would ruin your enjoyment of the candy, then the hallway is a logical place for you to eat it.

The same holds true of other unusual places people choose for eating, even if the selection was based on fear, apprehension, embarrassment, or any other such basically protective reaction.

Simply telling people to stop having such feelings, to free themselves and become uninhibited, self-assured eaters, is almost as naive as the diet organizations' approach of telling people to rigidly follow a prescribed regime like obedient little schoolgirls.

We remember a cartoon some years ago in which a psychologist slams his fist on the desk and shouts at a frightened little man, "Relax, damn it." We don't think it makes sense to shout at people that they "should" relax about their eating or "slow down," "eat less," "avoid 'poisonous' foods like chocolate and cheese." We very much discourage people from doing the same thing to themselves — that is, "making themselves" eat freely. Making someone else, or yourself, do anything is the antithesis of real freedom and won't work. The obvious proof with overeating is the persistence of obesity.

Sometimes someone at our workshops initially misinterprets the freedom to eat as a duty to eat "freely." We put the word "freely" in quotes, because in fact a person doing that is only substituting one kind of regimentation for another.

THE SECRET PEANUT-BRITTLE FIEND

There was, for instance, an early fortyish salesman who described himself as a "peanut brittle fiend." He never ate the candy where anybody he knew could see him, but consumed it by the bagful while driving along the highway, in motel rooms when he was on the road, and in his basement workshop when the rest of the family was busy upstairs.

Chris was very receptive to the idea that, even though he was sixty pounds overweight, he was entitled to pleasure himself with candy. So the very next weekend he took a huge bag of peanut brittle to a football game and ate it where his teenage son and a whole group of his own friends could observe him.

He felt sheepish and guilty about this, but he had formed the idea that he had to stop being ashamed of his candy eating and that he had to bring it out into the open, even if he wasn't hungry for it at the time.

The surprised comments and the teasing he got ruined his enjoyment of the football game, and he derived little pleasure from the candy. He was trying to eat defiantly, but was not in touch with himself.

We have talked of people who eat in unusual places because they are "undercover," or hiding. But, as we mentioned briefly, there is also a large group of people who do this sort of eating for a totally different reason: They genuinely enjoy eating that way; it fills a real need for them. Unfortunately, they often feel that this "out of the way" eating is aberrant and should be changed.

One such person was Ingrid, a statuesque, five-foot-ten, twenty-six-year-old blond from Minnesota who now works in a bank in Peoria, Illinois.

Ingrid claimed that her excess weight (which was only about ten pounds, but concerned her greatly) was strictly connected to the weather. In good weather, she came home from work, took a shower, put on shorts or jeans, and was off again for swimming or tennis or a walk. But on cold and rainy days she liked to fix herself a bath with lime-scented bath oil and luxuriate in the tub for up to an hour.

"The trouble is, while I'm drawing the bath water, I am fixing my tub snack. I know I sound like some self-indulgent Near-Eastern princess, but I just love to soak in that scented, oily water and sip and nibble."

On some days the snack consisted of a couple of Danish pastries and a big mug of Constant Comment tea; sometimes it was cookies and tea, and sometimes a glass of red wine and "some solid tasty stuff — a few smoked sprats, some boiled ham, a handful of olives, cheese . . ."

It took Ingrid some time, but she finally was able to view her bathtub eating as a pleasure she deserved.

The sensuous comfort of the warm water, combined with a pleasing scent and the deliberate tasting of some favorite foods and drinks, met a real need for her. It made her feel all right about herself and about the cold, rainy day. Psychologically, the bathtub is the ideal eating place for her. Her real difficulty was feeling compelled to eat a balanced dinner at 6:30 P.M., even when she was not at all hungry. Once she could accept eating dinner in the bathtub on rainy days, she began to lose weight.

Check yourself out for a moment:

(1) Where would you like to eat your favorite food?

(2) Where do you generally eat it?

If the answers to these two questions are not the same, try to focus on how to arrange your life so the two coincide more often. Would you derive greater satisfaction from these foods if you did eat them in the place where you would like to eat them? Or would there be so many interferences, from your own feelings and other people, that all enjoyment would be gone?

Ponder that for a while, then move on to another question: Assuming that you eat your reward food in one of the many "unusual" places, would it make you feel more satisfied and fulfilled to eat that food at a more conventional place like the dinner table, or at your desk, or off the coffee table while chatting with friends? Or would you feel cheated if you had to eat that food in one of these settings?

Picture it in your own mind. How would it be? Good? Bad? Unimaginable?

If you would feel cheated if you ate that food elsewhere, then the unusual place definitely is the place for you to eat.

In their advertising restauranteurs often make as much of the atmosphere of their establishments as they do of the cuisine. Psychologically speaking, they are right. A steak served in a tastefully decorated room at a table set with attractive china and linen and served by a pleasant, attentive waiter simply is not the same as a steak half pushed into your face on a chipped plate on a greasy table by a grouchy, short-tempered waitress in a food-splattered apron.

It doesn't taste the same, it doesn't please you the same, it doesn't give you anywhere near the same satisfaction. It feels distasteful even as we write these words! You might very possibly feel pleasantly full after that steak at the attractive restaurant and still have a hungry "I-want-some-thing-else" feeling after eating it at the greasy spoon.

NO LOBSTER, THANK YOU

David, a forty-eight-year-old black pharmacist from New Orleans now living in a suburb of Detroit, told us that there was something he couldn't understand. He was inordinately fond of shellfish, especially lobster, "But when you are raising six kids and want to send them to college, lobster just doesn't have much place in the family budget."

On a recent flight to a conference in Los Angeles, he had been delighted to find Maine lobster on the menu.

"I even said to my seat mate, 'Man, if they serve lobster, I'll fly their friendly skies anytime."

"And then I had a couple of martinis — and you know I like those — and then came that lobster, and I just couldn't enjoy it. Don't get me wrong. There was nothing wrong with the lobster; it was perfectly all right. But I simply couldn't enjoy it."

We talked some more of the flight, and eventually David himself saw the answer: He was deeply suspicious of airplanes and had been apprehensive about flying all his life. It was "irrational and childish," but he still couldn't shake the fear. In that atmosphere, he could not enjoy anything, not even lobster. The plane was not a safe place for him, and he got in touch with how necessary a feeling of safety was to his enjoyment of food.

"The best meals I've ever had," he mused "were in some pleasant little restaurants, all by myself."

He looked forward to family meals, but when he reviewed his eating patterns, he realized that he would be happiest to sit with his family at dinner time and have a drink and then eat later, by himself; enjoying food to the fullest was tied to solitude. This was a vital insight for David — knowledge that eventually helped him toward a freer eating pattern and weight loss.

David's case is not at all unusual. Many persons genuinely enjoy food most when they are alone. Others enjoy some meals with company, but need to eat alone at certain times. This has nothing to do with the obese person who eats alone because he dare not eat in other people's presence (a situation we discussed earlier). This is a person to whom eating alone isn't a lonely thing at all, but a prerequisite to gaining maximum psychological benefit from eating, an opportunity to experience all the nuances and subtleties of taste and aroma without interference.

Nancy, a thirty-eight-year-old mother of five children ranging in age from four to seventeen, felt her problem was night eating. "I don't just snack," she told the workshop group, "I dig in and eat."

She even went to the trouble of heating up leftover gravy and vegetables. "And believe, me, I make sure there always are leftovers when I cook!"

As she explored her attitudes toward food and eating, Nancy came to realize that these late-night meals, which she had in her bedroom after the children were asleep, were the only times when she actually tasted and experienced food.

"For all I know, I could be eating anything at the dinner table. It all tastes good, of course, but it just never satisfies me," she said. Yet the very same food, warmed over and eaten off the night stand with her feet propped up on the bed, was "great stuff. I'm really a pretty good cook."

Nancy could and did enjoy a restaurant meal with her husband and maybe one other couple, but the pressure of her duties as mother, the serving of the food, and the babble of conversation were too much for her. They not only lessened her food enjoyment; they actually deprived her of the ability to taste. So she began to just nibble at the dinner table. Her bedroom, she realized, was the right place for her to eat — not every night, but perhaps frequently. Nancy initially feared that she would set a bad example and pattern of eating for her children: "Imagine a four-year-old eating spaghetti on his bed!"

But she found that, after sufficient explanation, the children accepted that private eating is a personal need of hers, much as a before dinner cocktail is an adult prerogative, a specific taste. The children also soon realized that their mother was able to give them much more attention when she felt good about herself. She kept them company at the dinner table, drinking a glass of wine to relax but waiting to enjoy her own dinner later.

SHOULD YOU EAT AT YOUR OWN PARTIES?

Many other women can enjoy ordinary, everyday meals with their families, but not holidays or "company" meals. "It was frustrating for me to eat at my own dinner parties," said Carol, a Chicago suburbanite with a reputation as an excellent hostess. "No matter how hungry I am, when I'm hostess I have amnesia afterward about what I've eaten at the dinner table. I'm too busy and preoccupied to really taste and enjoy my food. Sure, it'll taste O.K. but after everyone leaves I have to eat again." Carol got insight into the fact that she engaged in amnesia eating under certain circumstances (at her own parties). Then the eating experience was wasted, and so she began to eat only token amounts. To her surprise, her guests rarely noticed.

Another woman volunteered, "I don't know why I even do it! Fixing that Thanksgiving turkey with all the trimmings, and serving it up prettily, and making sure the gravy stays warm and the rolls don't burn, and everything else, is such a hassle that I can't taste my food. When it's time to sit down at the table, all I really want is another old-fashioned. That would hum to me!"

Has anything like that happened to you? Have you found food tasteless because of circumstances and setting? Have you ever been to a cocktail party where you ate a lot of hors d'oeuvres, but afterward you couldn't tell what had been served because you really hadn't experienced any of it? Have you ever eaten dinner and then soon after wanted to eat again because, psychologically, you were still hungry?

One of our workshop participants had a startling experience last fall when his son entered first grade. It helped the father to clarify one of his own eating problems. "You know, Mike is a bright kid," he explained to us, "but every evening when I ask him, 'What did you have for lunch today?' he just mumbles something about, 'I forget, I think it was spaghetti.' Now you know damn well they don't have spaghetti every day. But why can't he remember what he ate?"

Then Mike woke up one night with a frightening dream. He had dreamed that he was lying on the cafeteria table and all the children and teachers were there, laughing and jeering at him.

After this dream he was able to tell his parents how scary a place the cafeteria was to him, with its high noise level, children pushing and shoving, and everything still so new and different to him. Mike couldn't tell his father what he had for lunch because he, too, couldn't remember the experience of the food. Like Carol, he was involved in amnesia eating.

The emotional factor of safety may be involved in eating, as it was for David and young Mike. Some may speculate that this is ancient and primitive "race knowledge." It may go all the way back to Pleistocene man who had to drag a killed animal to a safe place if he didn't want some predator (or the big fellow from the next cave) to take it away from him. But then again, it may only go back to your kid brother who could snitch a big chunk of icing off your cake while you weren't looking.

All such explanations, historical or very personal, may have validity, but the way you feel and react now is what's important. And many people have a strong, legitimate need for privacy *now* while eating and need to respond accordingly.

Jack Shelton, who puts out *The Private Guide to Restaurants in San Francisco* and spends his life sampling restaurants all over this country and abroad, made an interesting statement on his radio program. Talking about what kind of setting makes for a successful restaurant, Shelton pointed out that nobody ever seems to want "that big table in the middle of the room." People much prefer to sit in a booth, he claims, or at a table that has some sort of feeling of privacy, or even just against the wall. He said he could sum up the feeling people want in a restaurant in one word: "womb-like."

That interesting observation from a bona fide gourmet might be reassuring to those who like to take a bite of something with their head below window level in their car, or in the pantry with the door closed, or in the office elevator.

We feel that Shelton's use of the word "womb-like" is "psychologizing." The "back to the womb" syndrome has been talked and written to death by too many amateur and pseudopsychologists. We do agree with his basic premise that the majority of people prefer a feeling of privacy, if not actual privacy, for their dining. It is not a need restricted to overweight people. In many cultures — notably in Asia and Polynesia — eating is not considered a social activity, but rather a private affair.

DOES CONVERSATION MIX WITH FOOD?

Aside from a desire for privacy or safety, conversation is an integral part of an enjoyable meal for some people. To others, it's a distraction from the primary business at hand: eating and drinking. (Professional wine tasters never engage in conversation beyond the briefest remarks while tasting. They want to savor and experience their wine fully.)

Neither approach — mixing food and conversation, nor keeping them separate — is right or wrong. There simply are social eaters and solitary eaters. And many people find themselves in either category at different times, depending on mood and other variables.

The solitary eater is sometimes called antisocial or withdrawn or inhibited or selfish or rude. None of these labels is justified unless that person is antisocial or inhibited or whatever *in addition to* or *quite aside from* being a solitary eater.

For liberated eating, a person needs to know what his own preferred manner of eating is and then try to arrange his life accordingly. Too often obese people invalidate or criticize their own eating-style preferences and assume that they are not entitled to the particular food or locale that is most pleasurable. A "thinny" has no difficulty seeking out food pleasures, eating in a liberated way and maintaining a slender body. Fatties are not supposed to give reign to their preferences, and so lose touch with their inner needs.

For some people it is agreeable and even essential to mix several pleasurable experiences together; others enjoy them singly, one by one.

Check yourself out on these important variables: How do I like to eat, alone or in the company of others? At all times, or only sometimes? Whose company is desirable? Or is it only tolerable? And whose company is intolerable? When is eating companionship desirable? Or tolerable? When is it intolerable?

Serious disturbances in a person's relationship to food and in the whole eating pattern can result from not being aware of these needs and/or not meeting them.

Contemplate for a moment how often you have heard someone say, "I shouldn't have eaten all that," and how often you yourself have felt that way, feeling stuffed or bloated rather than comfortably full.

Try to re-create, in your mind, the last time that occurred. And the time before, and other times, if you can.

Did you eat "the whole thing" because it was such an enjoyable experience that you just couldn't bring yourself to interrupt it, even though your stomach was sending you a "full" signal? Or were you not really aware of eating that much because you were talking to someone, or listening, or both? Or were you reading a book or a newspaper, or watching TV, or listening to the radio? Did you more or less automatically eat the food till there was no more on the plate and the "unit" was finished?

We want to dispel quickly any idea that we are advocating solitary eating as a means of weight control. This is no more our intention than it is to make slow or fast eaters out of people, or to turn them on to or off any specific foods. But in our experience overeating often results from not recognizing, ignoring, or condemning such legitimate needs as privacy.

The opposite can happen just as well: The social eater who is forced to eat in solitude may overeat, or gobble food just to finish it.

THE FAMILY THAT WASN'T THERE

When Rosa signed up for a workshop, she brought along her wedding picture: a lithe, doe-eyed girl of nineteen with cascading black hair, a true Italian beauty. She was now twenty-nine, her eyes squinting out over bulging cheeks, her waist undistinguishable under a snug-fitting size 22 1/2 dress.

"It's the divorce that did it," she said. "Ever since the divorce I have just kept gaining and gaining. I don't think it's ever going to stop until I'll explode some day, or maybe my heart will give out."

Rosa found some quick comfort in the workshop simply from the camaraderie that develops. Seeing other people just as heavy as herself, or heavier, and hearing them talk frankly about their food problems was a reassuring experience to her. The aspect of Rosa's relationship to food that is pertinent in the present context boils down to this: Rosa came from a large, warm, close-knit New York Italian family, where everybody gathered for meals in the kitchen, always including some grandparents, aunts, uncles, or second cousins, as well as the immediate family.

When we asked Rosa to randomly name some images, smells, feelings that came to her mind when she thought of meals at home, she closed her eyes and came up with: "Big, steaming pots of soup. Pasta shining with butter. Aunt Sophia grating cheese. Mushrooms frying in butter. A gigantic pot roast in a pan about as big as a washtub. Mama with her wire whisk in hand saying, 'No bothering me now children. You want the zabaglione to get curdled?' Dad pouring wine from a big jug. Helping Mama put the filling in zeppole di San Giuseppe [St. Joseph's Day creampuffs] and then getting to lick the bowl."

After her marriage, Rosa moved to Hammond, Indiana. She loved her husband, George, but she did miss her extended family, even though she had two cousins with their families living nearby. They shared all holiday meals and many others besides.

After not quite eight years of marriage George left Rosa and their then six-year-old son because, he said, he longed to try a different lifestyle — with a different woman. This was a tragedy for Rosa. Not only did she love George, but there had never been a divorce in her whole family. ("Grandma back in Italy still doesn't know about it.")

The Hammond cousins were kind to Rosa and tried to make her and the boy feel as welcome as before. But she felt that she was the black sheep, the relative they had to be ashamed of. So when the trucking firm she worked for opened an office in the San Francisco Bay area, Rosa applied and got a job there. She took an apartment in one of the smaller communities on the east side of San Francisco Bay.

Her whole lifestyle changed. Only one thing hadn't changed, and this is something she had been unaware of until she began to explore it in the workshop: Rosa was still cooking for a large family, even though there was hardly ever anybody except her little boy to share a meal with.

She was still cooking big pot roasts — "not as big as Mama's, but I guess they are big" — making large batches of pasta, big pots of soup, and chicken *cacciatore* and bowls of zabaglione.

"Well, you can't make zabaglione with one egg!" she said somewhat defensively. But by the time she was saying this, she had already taken one giant step. She had come to realize that, regardless of the antecedent reasons, her overeating was based on her desire to recreate a warm, social eating and living atmosphere. And even though she would feel quite miserable eating huge meals with only her son for company, they afforded her comfort and a feeling of security.

Having gotten in touch with her emotional use of food, Rosa tried to tune in to humming foods and concentrate just on those, rather than dishes she cooked merely out of habit. She discovered that she really didn't care whether or not she had zabaglione and the many other elaborate desserts she had been preparing. The chicken dishes were unimportant, and, to her great surprise, even pasta hummed only once in a while. The foods she really craved to cook, to smell, and to eat — because all three of these elements were important to her — were the soups, the pot roasts, and the breads.

Rosa has not become the lithe, doe-eyed beauty yet. She may never regain her girlhood figure. But her weight stabilized with liberated eating, and then started a very slow descent. When we last saw her (she was bringing us a *corona di Nove*, a special Easter bread), she was wearing a size 14½.

WHAT ABOUT THE BUDGET?

At this point, you may fear that there will be a discrepancy between what you want (what hums) and what you can afford. Stop for a moment to assess your past battle record. How much money and energy have you been expending for your warfare with weight and food? Have you spent money on diet pills, medical visits, weight-losing organizations, or dietetic foods? Can you visualize spending that money on pleasurable foods instead? If you have a weight or food problem, buying humming foods can be viewed almost as a medical expense. Can you accept the view that treating yourself is a medical necessity? We believe that it is.

Speaking of economy, what about your own total economy of living? How much of your life — how much of your potential for enjoyment — is being squandered while you keep yourself in a straitjacket of dieting, calorie-counting, and jailbreak binging? We're concerned about the long-range economy and joy of living.

Getting in touch with your own feelings about where and how you eat is an essential part of establishing a relaxed, satisfying, stable relationship to food.

We suggested earlier that you try and picture in your own mind *where* you would like to eat. Now, try to picture how you would like to eat dinner, in terms of the best possible combination of all factors.

Picture a food or combination of foods that make up an enjoyable dinner for you. It doesn't matter whether that's steak and baked potato, or pasta, or mince with mealy dumplings, or stuffed sour-sweet cabbage — whatever appeals to you.

Got the image in your mind? Can you smell it? Can you anticipate the taste?

Now consider for a moment: Where is this food in your imaginary eating situation? Is it on a well-set table? At home? In a restaurant? In your bedroom? On a counter top?

In your imagination, are you sitting down, and if so, where? Or are you standing up? Or lying down? Were you automatically assuming that you would be sharing this meal with others, or was this occasion something for you alone? If people were there, who are they?

Think about the answers to these questions for a while. Compare this imaginary meal setting to the circumstances under which you usually eat your meals. Do they match? If not, is there anything you can do about it?

This is another situation where awareness of needs and preferences often leads to change. Many people don't eat under the circumstances most conducive to genuine food enjoyment because they haven't focused on their own needs. You might try a few experiments to put yourself in touch with your real desires and preferred food situations.

Those who usually eat with others have an easier time here than those who usually eat alone. As in the case of Rosa, they may not be eating alone by choice, and it may be difficult or even impossible for them to change this reality. If this is where you are — a social eater involved in solitary eating by circumstances — try nevertheless to determine how you can give yourself the optimal enjoyment.

To start with, do you usually eat sitting down or standing up? Stand-up eating is perfectly legitimate for some people, and they have a good feeling about it. Others prefer to keep a plate on the kitchen counter and eat their food bite by bite while keeping busy with some other activity, because it isn't worth the bother to them to set the table.

Also, stand-up eating does not seem like a commitment to manage a real meal. So, a person often feels that such food intake doesn't count. It's a way of fooling yourself when you're on a diet. You don't mean to eat; you're just having a bite. It's unofficial eating, usually unplanned or impulsive.

People who live with others and usually eat with others may also fall into this pattern. But we mention it in the context of solitary eating because it is most common among people who live alone, as is watching TV while eating.

FOR ON-THE-RUN EATERS

If you are one of these eaters, one of the on-the-run, on-the-lap, why-bother-for-just-me types, explore your relation to food with a few eating-awareness experiments.

For the next meal that you can eat without being rushed, set the table with a linen cloth or an attractive place mat — whatever you think you might enjoy. Have a cocktail first, if that is what you like. Then set out all the food, including your favorite beverage. Don't forget the salt and pepper, mustard or catsup or Worcestershire sauce if you like any of these. Bread and butter if you like them. A napkin. Flowers? Candles?

Now sit down and start to eat, slowly if that is enjoyable, fast if that is more your style. In either case, try to concentrate on the food. Don't read; don't turn on the radio or TV. Let your senses zero in on the food. Let your lips and tongue and teeth experience the food.

After you have eaten for a few minutes to satisfy physiological hunger, get up. Walk to the other side of the room. Look at a picture or gaze out the window for a few moments. Let your mind go blank if you can. Then focus on yourself.

Tune in to yourself and to the way you now feel. Be aware of the way your body feels as well as your psychological state at this point. Is there still a feeling of hunger? If so, where? In your gut, throat, lips? Or do these areas feel content? Some people feel annoyed at having had their meal interrupted. Others have a sense of contentment. Some experience anxiety about what will happen next. Others report a euphoric non-concern. Which kind are you?

Do you feel like going back to the table? Do you want to resume where you left off?

If you have good feelings about this leisurely way of eating, continue. If you have no bodily desire or yearning to take another bite, clear the table and put the rest of the food away.

But suppose you are in between; you want to eat more, but things aren't quite right. Something is missing. Turn on the radio or hi-fi to your favorite type of music, then resume eating. Is that more enjoyable?

EATING AND WATCHING TV

If it isn't, try reading or watching TV. What happens to food sensations now? Most people find that reading or watching TV so engrosses them that eating becomes mechanical and food is processed rather than experienced. But to some people, radio or TV are companionship or relaxing. They feel they would be giving up something pleasurable if they couldn't eat and read; or eat and listen; or eat and watch TV.

Phyllis was one of these people. She was a divorced legal secretary in her fifties. After a hard day's work, she loved to eat *and* read or watch TV. This to her was sheer pleasure: submerging herself in relaxing stimuli.

Phyllis tried to eat without any distraction. Her reaction: "I taste more, sure, but after a while I just get bored, and I end up feeling very dissatisfied."

What we told Phyllis was, "By all means, continue with what feels best. However, whether you are reading or watching TV, try to stick to light material while you are eating.

"Think of it this way: *You are creating a symphony of sensations* for yourself. The food is the virtuoso, the star performer, and you are the conductor. Your main attention belongs to the star. In fact, in many ways you are taking your cues from it. The other members of the orchestra are important. Beading can be your second violin, or TV can be the brass section, but they need to be modulated so they don't drown out the star."

Phyllis found that by giving food the starring role in her meals, she could open herself up to many new eating sensations and pleasures. She discovered that her customary meals were pretty boring and began to experiment with different tastes and textures. Instead of starting off with a wedge of lettuce with bottled dressing, as she had for years, she tried "some different overtures."

She began to derive surprising delight from some of the fancier canned soups, particularly black bean with sherry and consomme madrilène. And sometimes she made herself some quickie hors d'oeuvres, such as rye crisp with cream cheese and an anchovy, or sliced salami and pickled chili peppers.

She tried what she called "the little French restaurant bit," with fruits and cheeses after the main course, and discovered more fun in this, too. "Grapes and a piece of strong-smelling Brie that's so ripe it's almost runny — what a finale!"

Pleasuring herself with meals in this fashion, Phyllis found that she no longer had the same need for large quantities of food. By allowing herself the legitimate multi-sensory input of hors d'oeuvres, cheeses, and fruits she could savor foods and feel satisfied.

But these are other people's experiences and you'll want to explore for yourself exactly where you are. That is the important thing.

TO EAT IN OR OUT?

If you occasionally have the choice of eating at home or at a restaurant, check out this experiment: Try to eat a fairly identical meal under the circumstances you have found most agreeable at home, then at a restaurant. By "fairly identical" we do not mean that it has to be the exact combination of food, but something that is really humming to you on that particular day.

How does the total effect of home-eating compare to the restaurant-eating? Is the impersonal sociability of the restaurant a plus or a minus? Does preparing food add to your enjoyment, or is it far more satisfactory to have the food appear in front of you, ready to be eaten?

Check out the social eating situations that are available to you, such as eating at a club, at a church function, with friends or relatives, even at a community pancake breakfast. Often at such functions people hardly taste the food (though they may eat large quantities), because intense sociability gives them no chance to tune in to the food. Others enjoy the food and try to minimize contacts with other people, who represent an unwanted distraction. But to some, the combination of sociability and food is appealing, with one complementing the other.

If you feel you are part of the latter group, could you create more such eating situations for yourself?

Some people who live and eat alone are astonished to find that solitary eating, once they accept liberated eating, does actually give them the opportunity for intense food enjoyment. Previously they thought of eating alone as a drawback in their mode of living.

They may find that they have been focusing their loneliness on mealtimes and also bedtimes. These are the occasions that easily become symbolic of loneliness. Eating alone is a manifestation of living alone and therefore can become a time of sadness. We've often heard the statement, "I live alone and usually have to eat alone, but I simply don't enjoy eating without people." Our response is:

"What else can you do to pleasure yourself? A bath? A trip to the bakery? A small bottle of champagne? Remember you have the freedom to eat and also to not eat. If you don't enjoy eating alone, then why eat, other than to take care of hunger pangs?"

Other people who live alone tell us that they overeat because of their sadness. It's as if they're comforting themselves for the unhappiness of being alone. This was the problem of Sue, a widow in her fifties with all her children grown. She missed the liveliness and warmth and love of her family. They were gone, so she filled the empty meal table with sewing projects and snacked her way through the day. She felt she should keep busy and that feeling lonely was immature.

Sue found it helped her to plan her eating carefully. She wasn't alone; she had herself to take care of. Her loneliness was also the emptiness of not experiencing herself and her own feelings. She was on a diet to regulate not only food, but also her sadness and loneliness. She felt she *should not* have such negative emotions. We often find that people treat certain emotions as taboo and unacceptable, and thereby reject a valid part of themselves. This usually creates a gulf between who they genuinely are and who they wish they could be and that gulf is experienced as emptiness. It's as if the more people try to deny or suppress reality feelings (loneliness, sadness), the more intensely they feel empty, and need to use food as filler.

What about the opposite, the people who always eat with a family, or with others? To gain greater awareness of your needs, we suggest that you create an opportunity for eating a meal alone. Notice that we said a "meal." Almost everybody snacks alone at times, but a fork-and-knife meal is different.

This may seem impractical and selfish, but think of it this way: Your past battles with weight and food undoubtedly have created tension at mealtimes with your family (not to mention your meals with others). Once you become liberated from the rat-race of diets and conflict over taboo foods, you and everyone around you will benefit. You can explain to your family that you simply need the freedom to experiment.

Try exploring this idea of solitary eating. Go through the same steps outlined for the solitary eater, setting the table and exploring how you react to food in total solitude, or with music, or with light reading or TV viewing. If this is too difficult, explore alternatives. If you work and usually eat with friends or colleagues, try going out for a late lunch, after your usual eating companions have left. Go to a restaurant or coffee shop that you don't usually patronize and explore eating alone there, for a beginning.

Many people report that when they eat this way, the food seems to taste different. They may actually be tasting and experiencing some familiar foods for the first time, because in their customary eating patterns the taste sensations get overpowered by other sensory input inherent in a group eating situation.

Consider now the people you usually eat with. Do you ever watch them eating? How do you feel about their eating styles? People have a vast variety of reactions to seeing and hearing other people eat. With some people you may experience a warm, happy, compassionate, sharing feeling when you watch them eat. With others you may feel uncomfortable, as if you want to blank them out and neither look nor listen while they are eating. Some people's table manners may even disgust you, although you like the people otherwise.

Joan, the mother of two children aged three and five, reported that she sometimes felt nausea when she ate with her children and watched them eat. She realized that their style of eating was normal and expected for their age, but watching them slurp and drool and pick up food made it impossible for her to stay in touch with her own food and to find pleasure in it.

FOR MORE SENSUOUS EATING

Many nonverbal messages pass between people when they eat. So, even when there is minimal conversation, there can still be strong communication. Those who saw the movie *Tom Jones* undoubtedly remember the wordless eating scene, which may well be one of the most sensuous encounters ever put on film. Eating is sensuous, and it follows that you might give the choice of eating partners at least some of the attention that you give the choice of sex partners.

Next time you are eating with someone whose company you enjoy, you might try a few experiments.

First, eat in complete silence for a few minutes. How does it feel to experience the physical presence of another person and be aware of the mutual activity of eating, without any conversation?

Generally, in our society silence at meals occurs only in a tense or monotonous atmosphere: a couple, bored stiff with each other, sitting at a table silently processing food. Food then becomes a shield or barrier. In that case, the people are in touch with neither each other nor themselves. If anything, food is used by them as a buffer so they don't have to relate but have something to do.

We are suggesting the very opposite of this scene: a loving situation with nonverbal sharing and a deep awareness of the other's presence. Focus on the other person's enjoyment of food.

Can you *concentrate* on the enjoyment of food? Do you experience a sense of loneliness, or is there sharing on a different level of awareness? Do you enjoy your food? More than usual? Or less? Does the food taste different?

Next, put down your fork and knife and talk for a few moments without eating. Then resume eating, but without speaking. Try this sequence several times, alternating between eating silently and conversing without eating, rather than mixing them in the accustomed way. Which style is more comfortable? Which is disturbing?

When you have finished the meal during which you alternate food and conversation, stop for a brief evaluation.

How much did you eat? The same amount as usual? More? Less? How do you feel? Satisfied or still wanting something? Does this differ from the way you generally feel after a meal? How would you like to eat your next meal? All your meals?

THE MID-MEAL MEANDER

Midway through a meal, especially if you are at a restaurant, get up and walk to the bathroom for a few moments. We call this the "mid-meal meander." This is not rude, nor is it just a clever stratagem to make yourself eat less, though that sometimes happens. The mid-meal meander provides time to check out where you are. Are you full? Does something still hum to you? Is it comforting to know that there is food waiting for you?

Some of our workshop participants tell us that prior to coming to our Institute one of their major problems was, "Once I start eating a meal I can't stop until I'm stuffed." This happens because eating can become automatic. Many people tend to consider a meal finished only when all the food on the plate is gone. You may keep on eating just because there is food on the plate, without ever stopping to think whether you still want it. The mid-meal meander breaks up the automatic quality of eating, allowing you to assess yourself and the extent of your hunger. You can then make your choices.

The amount of food you eat should be determined only by you and how you feel, not by what someone else considers a serving. Restaurants especially tend to be overgenerous. The mid-meal meander is a way of getting in touch with yourself and we highly recommend it, whether you're at home, eating at a restaurant, being served on a plane, or dining out socially.

8/ *DON'T LET OTHERS PRESSURE YOU*

This is for people who get pressured by others and hassled about their eating or their weight. Even though others may mean to encourage you, the effect of their advice or warnings is usually to make an overweight person feel depressed, angry, or even more ravenous. Fortunately, there are ways to liberate your eating from the influence of friends, family, and dinner hostesses.

"Come on, you can go back on your diet tomorrow!"

"You don't have to be good *all* the time!" "Just a little bit won't hurt."

How often have you heard these phrases? Almost as often as "You really should go on a diet" or "You know, it really isn't good for your health to be so heavy?"

People who make such statements — and it makes little difference whether they are advising you to eat or to diet — usually are:

- insensitive and simply parroting platitudes;
- well-meaning, but invading your privacy;
- feeling threatened and negative toward you;
- self-righteous and feeling smug or superior;

- mothering you and feeling good about being helpful, maternal advice-givers.

We bring this topic up because interference from other people is often one of the biggest stumbling blocks to staying in touch with your body wisdom and losing weight.

We would like to cite some comments from people we have worked with. Can you identify with any of them?

"I feel good weighing less and eating what I dig. But my roommates keep telling me I looked better before. They say now I look weak and that my face is drawn."

"I feel I have the right to *not* eat when I'm full. But would you tell that to my mother on Thanksgiving?"

"Sure I believe that I have a right to eat what I want, but who is going to convince my husband?"

"What really hummed to me yesterday morning was butter-brickle ice cream with chocolate syrup. But how could I eat that in front of the children? They'd never eat their soft-boiled eggs again."

"All I wanted for lunch was a bourbon on the rocks and the dessert, but those other guys would've thought I was strange, or kidded me about being on another diet."

"The trouble is, Hank always brings home a treat for the kids and me Friday nights. So here was this gooey strawberry parfait cake . . ."

"My sister-in-law says losing weight has brought out all the wrinkles in my face."

"Jose thinks I'm fine the way I am. He insists I don't need to lose weight, even though I'm twenty-eight pounds too heavy."

"I wasn't really hungry, but Dad said it might be a hell of a long time before he would celebrate another promotion in a fancy place like this again."

"Jane is so proud of her gourmet cooking. If I'd told her that chicken *chausseur* just didn't hum to me, she'd have been hurt."

All this means that these people eat *what* they don't want or *when* they don't want to because they are allowing someone else to pressure them.

The two pertinent questions are:

(1) What is going on with other people when they make these "helpful" comments?

(2) What can you do about them?

WHY THEY PRESSURE YOU

You can deal with these pressures effectively if you can get in touch with the other person's motivations.

We stated at the outset that people who interfere with your eating may feel threatened by the success of others; they may feel negative toward you; or they may be thoughtless, or well meaning but insensitive.

In our society, almost every person wishes that he or she could modify or improve his or her life or behavior in some respect. Many would like to manage their time better so they wouldn't always feel they are behind schedule. (Housewives suffer from a high incidence of this yearning and so do most professionals, male and female.) Others feel they should handle finances more effectively; or that they should improve their grooming; or do more to further their education; or should strive harder for professional success; or should learn to control their temper; or should be less inhibited in showing warmth and affection toward others; or should be more relaxed when speaking to a large group of people; or should be more active in politics and community affairs; or should learn how to converse with strangers at large parties; or should be better listeners; or should be more successful in sex.

Others feel they really should stop smoking; cut way down on drinking; stop wasting time watching TV; spend more time with the children; or exercise more. The list could go on and on.

In most instances, efforts to achieve these goals are hidden from the public's eye. Failure to "improve" one's behavior is usually known only to that person, unless he is a chain smoker or an alcoholic. (And even the alcoholic can frequently hide his addiction.)

The overweight person has no such privacy. His eating — or not eating — is generally open to the scrutiny of family and friends. Certainly his gaining or losing weight is a matter of public view. So what happens when you become successful? What is the reaction when you start to lose weight, especially if you're not on any of the usual torturous, self-depriving diets, and are eating as freely as a "thinny"?

ARE THE OTHERS JEALOUS?

It can be an uncomfortable challenge to the rest of us who have not managed to modify our behavior in whatever our main area of concern is. *You're winning your battle while we may make no dent in what we want to change.*

For example, Norma, a mid-thirtyish nurse we worked with, got some very strong critical reactions from her husband when she got within ten pounds of her desired weight. (She had been thirty pounds over that.)

"I can't figure out what's gotten into Neil," she told us. "For years he's been after me to lose weight, telling me that a nurse especially should know better than to endanger her health with all those extra pounds.

"Now it's the very opposite. He tells me he doesn't like skinny women, as if I were Twiggy! He says I don't fix his favorite foods anymore, when I am really having fun cooking for the first time in years. I'm stumped."

It took a little detective work to find what was bothering Neil. He was a passionate sweets eater and a heavy smoker. He also had a moderate drinking problem. He had been trying to battle these three habits for years with little success. So long as Norma was overweight, he didn't feel threatened; she hadn't succeeded either. Now he was afraid that she would ultimately confront him with "Look at me! I managed, so why can't you?"

Norma was not a self-righteous person and would probably never have made such a statement. But within himself Neil felt his own failure more acutely because of her success, and his resentment found an outlet in putting her down, deriding her success and even making something negative out of it.

This is a very common, very human, very understandable reaction. Husbands especially often feel threatened by their wives' weight losses. (Other men might get interested in her, and she in other men.)

One of the comments earlier in this chapter was from a woman who told her sister-in-law, Helen, that getting thin had brought out the wrinkles in her face. These two women had never had a warm relationship, but had tried to get along as a matter of family courtesy. Helen kept her home attractive and her children well-dressed, and was an excellent cook. Yet she felt incompetent as a person because of her weight.

Her sister-in-law was highly competitive. She was a rather poor homemaker, but so long as Helen was fat the sister-in-law could feel she was ahead. She felt more competent as a woman. Her snide comment to Helen about wrinkles showed that she wished Helen would go back to being fat. It would make *her* happier.

Needless to say, the person who also has a weight problem can experience extreme feelings of envy or jealousy or frustration when someone else does the unimaginable: Losing weight *and* kicking the diet habit at the same time. He may go on the warpath, looking for anything to criticize, real or imagined, to get the other fattie back into the club.

In such cases, real viciousness is not uncommon — as in the case of the two young women who told their roommate that she was prettier when fat.

Your independence, your freedom to eat and not eat, may be a source of annoyance to others. A hostess knows in her heart that she should not urge overweight guests to take seconds. But she may consider it part of her role to urge people to eat more. That is what a good hostess should do. Also, for her self-gratification, she likes to see people eat all she has cooked. To her that represents recognition of her talents and her value.

If a hostess knows you've had a weight problem, she might add solicitously: "If you're on a diet, you can go back on it tomorrow." Or "Just this one time won't hurt you." Or "It really doesn't have all that many calories."

How do you respond when that happens to you? Many people tell us that they take "a little bit of everything to make the plate look full." Or they "just sort of mess up the plate, work the food around so it looks like I've eaten." Or they may take a bite whenever they think they are being watched.

These subterfuges may pacify the hostess, but the overweight person feels uncomfortable and eventually angry — usually at himself. Invariably, the person gets out of touch with himself and his body wisdom. Very often he gets a frustrated "the hell with it" feeling and abandons himself to food, overeating without gaining pleasure or satisfaction.

When such negative events happen inside a person, it is bound to affect his relationship with his hostess and other guests. It tends to ruin the social as well as the culinary aspect of the evening.

We have found it best to prevent such situations at the outset.

HOW TO HANDLE A HOSTESS

Suppose you have come to a party but aren't hungry; or you arrive and nothing is humming to you. You might tell your hostess: "I'm troubled about something, but I'm afraid to tell you because I hate to disappoint you." The thoughtful hostess will say just what you would probably say in the same spot: "Please tell me. Whatever it is, it won't offend me."

Then you have the perfect opening for saying, "I hate to admit it, but I'm just not hungry tonight." And the good hostess really has no other out than to tell you, "That's perfectly all right. I'm glad you came anyway."

Another good opener is to say, "I almost telephoned to say I couldn't come because I'm not hungry tonight. But I decided to come anyway because I enjoy seeing you."

One middle-aged bachelor, charming and outgoing, found the perfect answer for the really overbearing hostess, the one who won't take "no" for an answer, no matter what: "I just say in a slightly ominous voice, 'I really do have to be careful, you know. I have a potassium deficiency.' It works beautifully. Nobody knows what the hell a potassium deficiency is, but nobody wants to admit their ignorance. So they leave you alone."

WHEN CHILDREN OBJECT

Objections to your weight change and your different eating pattern within the family are a different matter.

Children sometimes feel threatened by a change in a parent. If Mommy or Daddy has always been fat and suddenly isn't, the child often wonders what else might change in his world. He may worry that the parent's love and concern for him, or all sorts of comfortable and familiar habits of family life, might change as well.

If something as familiar as Mommy's body size can change, all sorts of unknown happenings may occur. The stable, predictable parts of life may not be safe, either.

Parents, especially mothers, have often told us of their puzzlement when their young child says, "You're not fat, Mommy. You're soft. Don't you change."

Apprehension in the child is especially common when the parent's new eating pattern includes such strange novelties as Mommy eating alone in her bedroom sometimes or Daddy sitting at the dinner table with nothing but a cup of coffee or a glass of wine or a drink in front of him. Or a parent might refuse to share a box of candy, saying, "You can have your own box of candy. This one is mine. I really need this all to myself."

It is important for parents to be aware of these possibilities so they can reassure children. You might point out to a child that his own body keeps changing, but that this does not influence the loving relationship in the family. You might show him pictures of himself as a baby and toddler and tell him how happy you were when he was born. Then you might say, "Look at yourself now, how much bigger you are and how different you look. But I am just as happy that you are mine, and I love you just as much as when you were younger."

Stop now for a moment and think about all the people who make comments about your eating: the ones who, over the years, lectured you on the dangers of overweight and advocated weight-losing schemes; who came up with critical and cautionary remarks when you did lose weight; who are now openly hostile or sarcastic if they have observed a change in your eating pattern and your approach to food since you started reading this book.

IT'S THEIR PROBLEM, NOT YOURS

If you are like the majority of overweight people, you have spent a lot of time wondering what is wrong with you, what is the reason for your dysfunctioning, especially after you have listened to "helpful" people.

Consider the possibility that your eating — or the change that has occurred in it — often touches on painful problems in other persons. It may be psychologically sound and valid from their own perspective to say the things about you that they say. But then it's their problem, not yours. You have a right — indeed, you owe it to yourself — to recognize the problem as such, and to put things into the correct perspective.

If someone is upset and angered by observing that you are eating freely — that you're not eating because you are not hungry, or because you are gaining or losing weight — *that's their problem.*

Focus on the fact that their behavior toward you is motivated by their own hang-ups and is irrelevant to you, so there is no point in letting it influence you.

If the person making these remarks is someone you care for, you may want to help him with his problem. You won't help him by accepting the put-down. So what are you to do? We believe that it is important to do something right when it happens. It is important for you. Because even if you pretend to ignore them, these "innocent" comments can have adverse effects on you.

For example, a young girl with whom we later worked was stopped by a priest in the street. "Excuse me, young lady," he said, "do you realize you're damaging your health with your weight and that you simply must go on a diet?"

She felt fury rising inside herself, yet she thanked him for his concern. Then she went home and went on a memorable eating binge that lasted almost three days. This may be an extreme example, but any comment about your body and your eating has an effect on you. And it is rarely helpful.

If a friend expresses what you believe to be genuine concern, how do you feel? Does it help you? Or do you still feel as though your autonomy and independence are being intruded upon?

In most people, these remarks produce, first, a feeling of humiliation; then anger and rebelliousness. Quite often the result is heavy eating, if not outright binging. The fact that you are being treated like a child frequently triggers a deep depression, and food may be the only comfort available to you. It's your way of going home and licking your wounds.

HOW DO YOU REALLY FEEL ABOUT MEDDLERS?

Overweight people often think they have become immune to such assaults on their integrity because they have come to expect them. That's like a black thinking he is immune to discriminatory behavior by whites. The hurt and the fury may be suppressed, but they are smoldering under a calm exterior.

Get in touch with what happens inside you when people make meddling remarks about your eating, your body and your weight. How did you react the last time? And what was your inward response — what did you do?

Basically, when you are subjected to such comments, three options are open to you:

- Go on the defensive and explain yourself (which pretty much amounts to entering a guilty plea).
- Launch a counterattack.
- Remove yourself from the ball game by stating or implying that your body and your eating are off-limits.

Which one you choose is a personal matter. It depends on what is comfortable for your own personality style. It also depends on the individual you are dealing with and the situation where the encounter takes place. The same person might choose different approaches at different times.

Jerry, a college physics instructor in his early thirties, had used mostly defensive humor when people told him he should lose weight. He had countered with something like "Hey, there's a thought." Or "I'd never noticed."

Sometimes he assured them, "You're absolutely right. Dieting has high priority on my list of projects. It's Number Eight." At times, especially with older people, he skipped the humor and said things like "Well, you know it runs in my family." Or "All of us Scandinavians are big-boned." Or "Didn't you know? I have a slight thyroid imbalance."

When Jerry finally felt liberated in his eating and was losing weight, he still received static from some people. Some of it came from his mother, who could not comprehend his new relationship to food and the whole underlying philosophy. So what he told her, in essence, was this:

"Mom, you know how many diets I've tried, and you know what usually happened. In the long run — nothing. I think I finally straightened out my feelings about food. It might not be your way, but it's mine. It has to do with my body, and I feel good about it. So from now on, that's my private matter.

"I don't argue with you about the way you vote; I won't allow you to argue with me about the way I manage my body. This subject is no longer open for discussion. My eating is totally my responsibility."

With his girlfriend he used basically the same approach — declaring his weight and eating off-limits — but in a more sharing and tender way. He explained to her that he had very strong feelings about being told what to eat and what not to eat. He pointed out that she respected his integrity in other ways, so why not in this aspect of living? He reported that she felt quite embarrassed and told him she was sorry that she had been so insensitive. She had simply never thought about it in this way, but could accept the validity of his approach.

When still another person, a bright, smart-ass student in his informal senior seminar, commented, "Hey, I thought you were on a new get-thin kick. When are you going to stop feeding your face with pie?" Jerry used approach No. 2: counterattacking.

He said, "When are you going to stop masturbating?" Obviously Jerry would never have used such a blunt, earthy retort to his mother or girlfriend. Some people could never comfortably do it with anyone. But for those for whom this is possible, an analogy to sexual matters is often very effective.

IT'S LIKE SEX

Sex and elimination are intimate personal body matters, and most people respect them as such. Food and eating are also intimate personal body matters, but many people don't think of them this way.

You can point out to a friend that he or she would be highly offended if you asked, "Have you had any good sex lately?" or "When was your last orgasm?" Then you can explain that, for you, a question such as "Are you really going to keep those pounds off this time?" or "Do you still eat all that junk food?" is such an invasion of privacy.

In our advanced workshops we often discuss such experiences. Most people report that the people with whom they have real rapport generally respond well to "I appreciate your interest and concern, but I feel that my eating and my body are personal matters, and I'd rather not discuss it," or a brusque "Look, I like you, but this is simply none of your damn business." The latter (counterattack) method is generally useful against someone who is especially thick-skinned or a friend with whom you are so comfortable that you don't have to pull punches.

Linda, a twenty-eight-year-old supermarket checker, used this approach with her roommate, whom she had known and liked for three years.

"When she asked me, 'When are you going to do something serious about your weight?' I finally said, 'Did you have a good bowel movement this morning?'" The roommate got the point.

The majority of people with whom we have worked have found no benefit in trying to explain their new philosophy of food liberation and psychological insights to all askers. Many feel the urge to share their newfound freedom with friends and family members. They want to talk about how good it is to rejoin the joyous world of food after having been imprisoned in the dreary jail of diets and calorie-counting. They feel good about themselves, and they want others to know it. And then they encounter the "buts" — " *But* is it going to last?" "*But* are you getting proper nutrition?" "*But* eventually you have to find a more stable pattern." " *But* you can't go through life just eating what you want." "*But* the novelty will wear off and you'll be right back where you started." And on and on and on.

We'll let Derek, a pre-medical student, tell what happened to him: "At first, I just repeated it all again and said, 'Man, you just weren't listening to me.' But they came right back with more objections, so we started discussing and arguing, and I got myself all turned around saying things I didn't mean to say.

"I felt myself getting frustrated and angry. And then I suddenly stopped because this was crazy. I *was* right back where I started. I mean, here I was practically apologizing. I was allowing people to meddle in my life again. My body and my eating were being taken apart like some stiff on the dissecting table, and I was letting people do this.

"So I just said, 'Look, let's just say it's my business and drop it.'" He refused to get into any more discussions about his eating after this.

Most people in our groups have had similar experiences and agree that they can discuss the matter in depth with only a few people with whom they have good rapport on most important things in their lives, people who will listen long enough to really comprehend what they are saying.

9/ *COPING WITH FESTIVE DAYS*
   AND ETHNIC WAYS

Food conventions have a tyrannizing effect, whether imposed by oneself or society. This chapter offers new options for people to whom holidays are a time for dreaded weight gain. It is also for those who feel frustrated — those who either avoid savory cultural or ethnic dishes because they are too fattening, or eat such dishes, not because they really want them but for ideological loyalty.

Christmas comes but once a year.

So do Hanukkah, the Feast of the Ascension, Chinese New Year, Thanksgiving, Passover, Easter, the Fourth of July, your dad's birthday, Cinco de Mayo, Labor Day, and Succoth. It adds up to a lot of days, and they can all be meaningful, keeping you in contact with your own heritage and your family. They are also times of peril for anyone trying to lose weight — especially if it's by deprivation dieting.

Think back to your dieting days. Were some of the festive times we mentioned (and others like them) the times when you fell off the wagon? They usually are. For these are the times when the social pressures for eating conformity become formidable — and when beckoning foods are abundant.

Holidays and special occasions are the times when dieters most often allow themselves out of jail, either on parole or in a breakout. And since most dieters believe that they are serving life sentences — that they will never be free men and women in the world of tantalizing foods — they usually go on a rampage of overeating, all the while feeling guilty.

How often, in the past, did you say to yourself, "Starting New Year's Day, I'll go back on my diet and stay on it this time," or "After this meal, I'll really be strict about my diet?" Viewing a particular meal as the last freestyle eating — we call it the "death-row dinner" — often results in people eating immense quantities, eating themselves into a stupor, into oblivion.

But what could one expect when there is a threat that "this is the last time?" Under such conditions, no thought is given to what hums. Instead there is a desperate attempt to store up: food, pleasure, sensations, memories. This behavior makes sense from a psychological perspective, because the person is really dreading the morrow and storing up appears logical.

A camel going off into the desert eats and drinks that way. Unfortunately, it doesn't work for people. Remembrance of yesterday's food pleasures does little to lessen today's deprivation. Often, the denial is even felt more acutely, especially when there is no "tomorrow." The death-row-dinner approach can turn the happiest holiday into a bad memory.

Have you ever allowed the bathroom scale to judge last evening's dinner? Or how good a vacation you've had?

In your new, liberated way of eating, there is no such thing as falling off the wagon or eating the last pleasurable meal ever. Yet, the lure of beckoning foods and the pressures to eat what everybody else is eating will still be strong on these special days.

TWO WAYS NOT TO EAT HOLIDAY FOODS

In our experience, two almost diametrically opposed situations arise when it comes to holiday and ethnic foods.

On the one hand, there is the person who has deliberately avoided the traditional foods of his cultural background or of national or religious holidays. This is done primarily because these special foods tend to have high caloric value. Or the food may be rejected along with religious and social customs that no longer seem pertinent; they may be tainted by association with an overbearing mother or a restrictive mode of living — considered unsophisticated or archaic.

People who reject certain culturally important foods are often depriving themselves of much pleasurable and psychologically important eating. They may be creating vast areas of frustration because the food really is humming to them.

On the other hand, other people eat traditional holiday or cultural foods, even though these foods fail to hum to them. They tend to eat them mostly, perhaps even solely, because of family and social pressures. Sometimes people eat these foods because they themselves look upon such eating as a way of getting in touch with their family or origins and breaking out of a plastic lifestyle that lacks identity.

These people, too, are not allowing their inner signals to get through. If you eat something because mother would be offended if you didn't, you are letting another person run your eating. Sometimes the desire to establish a closer cultural or family identity is what really hums to you and you eat the food as a prop, as a way of getting closer. The food tastes good (as almost all food does), but it's not satisfying and you usually overeat.

In our workshops we have dealt with many people for whom traditional foods led to unhappy eating. Often they reject the cultural food that hums to them when they overeat on beckoning foods.

Karl was one of a large group of German scientists and highly skilled technicians who came to this country immediately after World War II. Basically an apolitical person, he had held a good job under the Nazi regime because of his technical skills. His family had enjoyed certain privileges, such as large food allotments and good housing away from their bomb-ravaged hometown, Cologne.

He had a nagging feeling of guilt about this. And when he came to the United States — again because of his technical skills — he decided to make a clean break with the past. He became a super-American. He switched his culinary loyalties from sauerbraten to steak, from pan-fried *frikadellen* to barbecued hamburgers, from fruit tortes to doughnuts, from potatoes cooked in the skin to candied yams.

When we started working with Karl he was almost sixty pounds overweight and was quite worried about his high blood pressure.

THE RHINELAND HUMMED

To the first workshop eating-awareness session, Karl brought a bag of chocolate doughnuts and potato chips as his favorite taboo foods. What he got in touch with later was that he liked these foods well enough. "They are among my favorite foods in the American framework," he said. But what *hummed* to him wasn't in "the American framework" at all. The things that he truly craved were German, and, even more specifically, regional foods of the Rhineland. He had denied himself these foods for over twenty years because they were part of the past he had left behind. And the dish he most longed for, once he allowed his mental guards to come down, was something called *Himmel und Erde.*

"That means 'heaven and earth,'" he explained with a slightly embarrassed laugh. "The heaven is apples, and the earth is potatoes, and you cook them together and sort of mash them. My mother always served pan-fried meats with that, like liver or bratwurst or pork chops."

When Karl got home that night he asked his wife to put away the dinner she had prepared. He wanted to go to a special small German restaurant for dinner. The next day, Karl was beaming. "I had two orders of *Himmel und Erde*, and I didn't even want dessert or my usual bedtime snack. That was the most wonderful meal I've had in years. It was like coming home." His eyes brimmed with tears as he spoke.

Karl did not totally switch back to German foods. On some occasions he found typically American foods and food combinations humming to him. That happened, for example, on his birthday, when Erika, his wife, had planned a menu centered around roast goose with prune stuffing and red cabbage with chestnuts.

"That one wasn't easy," Karl reported later. "But I finally asked Erika if we could have that birthday dinner another night. Because what hummed to me that day were a couple of martinis and a tossed green salad with Roquefort dressing. I was too excited to be able to taste or enjoy any other foods."

Karl derived great pleasure and satisfaction from his own mélange of German and American dishes and found that he had less and less need for eating or drinking large quantities. He summed up his new pattern with the description of one Saturday afternoon and evening:

"Even when I was dieting, I always used to give myself Saturday night off. I'd drink a pitcher of martinis, a small one, and eat one of those economy-size bags of chips along with two or three containers of dip from the deli. And then dinner.

"Last Saturday I looked at my watch and thought, 'Martini time,' but then I stopped and asked myself, 'Do I *feel* like martini time?' and I didn't. That martini jug was beckoning, but that's all.

"So I sat back in my recliner and closed my eyes and tried to listen to my insides. And you know what came to me? Something I hadn't even thought about in years, but it's a favorite snack where I come from. A glass of nice, medium-dry white wine and dark bread with butter and cheese — something like some Dutch Gouda — and onion rings.

"And that's what I had Saturday. Three glasses of wine and two of those open-face sandwiches. It was so marvelous and so satisfying that I didn't feel like dinner or anything else that evening. So that's all I had."

Karl wrote on his follow-up questionnaire that he had lost seventeen pounds by eating only what he craved, and was still losing effortlessly.

CHECK YOUR CHILDHOOD

There are many variations on this theme of cutting oneself off from one's origins. Can you identify in any way with this problem? You might ask yourself a few questions: Am I now eating the same kinds of foods I ate in my childhood? Am I eating the foods grandmother used to fix?

If the answers are mostly "no," try to explore how you feel about this. Perhaps your grandmother was a lousy cook. But most grandmothers made food with substance, flavor, and taste. Are these foods not easily available? Have you grown to dislike them? Do they bring back unpleasant memories? Do you avoid them because they are too starchy? Have you forgotten about them?

We want to relate a few more examples that might aid you in getting in touch with your own feelings about cultural or ethnic foods.

Connie's parents were Armenian and she had lived with "millions" of aunts and uncles and cousins on a farm near Fresno in California's Central Valley. When she was eighteen she went off to college, where she majored in art and fashion design. When we met her she was thirty-two, an assistant buyer in the sportswear department of a large store, married to an accountant, and in constant fear of becoming "really fat, like my mother and all my aunts."

Connie was seven pounds overweight, yet she lived in daily dread of becoming fat and kept almost hourly track of her total calorie intake for the day. She said, "I have a food computer in my head, and can never switch it off."

She and her husband had a large circle of friends and did a good deal of partying and eating out. They all liked "sophisticated" foods, Connie said, "but of course I try to emphasize proteins." She despised "those dull diet foods."

What Connie became aware of in our workshop was that she truly liked some of those foods.

She still craved the sweet honey pastries of her childhood, but she also craved some of the foods she had brushed off as diet stuff: yoghurt and fresh fruits and vegetables. These foods had become tainted by their association with diets. It took Connie several weeks of avoiding anything that seemed like diet foods to realize that some of these were actually humming foods. This was especially true of yoghurt, a cultural food for Armenians, which her mother had always made herself.

Initially Connie wondered, "How am I going to convince anyone that I'm eating yoghurt because I like it and not because I'm dieting and have to?" She eventually realized that she felt proud of her Armenian background and wanted to share her heritage and food loves with friends. She has become relaxed about food, enjoys her meals and mealtimes, and has lost several pounds.

STANLEY DIDN'T TRUST HIMSELF

Stanley had fought a battle with his weight ever since he became an adult. When he came to our workshop, he had just lost thirty-five pounds and was within ten pounds of his "ideal" weight.

"But I'm terrified that I might put those pounds right back on. I've done it too many times before, and I don't trust me!"

Stanley was then forty-two. He was a social worker, active in politics — and a champion dieter. He had been on just about every diet we had ever heard about, and he kept a double set of food scales, calorie lists, and conversion charts, one at home and one at the office,

When we discussed eating patterns, Stanley told the group that he had been "the lousiest eater in the world when I was a kid. I was skinny my first two years and my mother had to stuff every bit into me. But she did stuff it into me! She still tries whenever she gets a chance. That's why I hardly ever visit her."

Stanley also described his mother as "the cartoon version of the Jewish mother. I should write a play about her. It would be the comedy hit of the year."

He tried to rationalize his avoidance of Jewish food. "Have you ever eaten anything tougher than a bagel or more bland than matzos?" he asked at one point. Later he derided Jewish food in general: "It's all loaded with calories and full of cholesterol."

After Stanley had had his first guided food fantasy (see chapter 16) he was visibly shaken. In the fantasy, he had found himself swimming in an enormous lake of chicken soup — and it was totally pleasurable.

"I was blowing at the tiny rounds of fat that swim to the top of the soup till I got them all together into one big glob. And then I balanced these huge matzo balls on my shoulders, and they were incredibly light, and then they would roll down my back. Finally, the soup seemed to be flowing right through me. I floated on my back and was completely saturated with the smell and the taste and the feeling of it. And it was so good!"

That night after coming home from the workshop Stanley did his own further eating-awareness exercises with chicken soup. He tasted it in tiny spoonfuls; he gargled with it; he swooshed it through his mouth and spat it out; he sucked some through a straw. He thoroughly explored chicken soup and got in touch with his own feelings about it. When he reported back Sunday morning, he was sure that "chicken soup hums to me. Of all things — Jewish penicillin!"

For Stanley, the foods that he really enjoyed had become linked with his domineering mother and a religion that was no longer meaningful to him. So he had cut himself off from foods he really desired and needed for fulfillment in his eating.

Karl, Connie, and Stanley avoided culturally relevant foods that hummed to them. Others may respond to such foods in the opposite manner, eating them even though they don't hum.

Michele came to a workshop when she was nineteen. She had gained twenty-three pounds during the previous year, her freshman year at college, and she hated every pound of it. The daughter of a black physician in Seattle, she had grown up in a "typical uptight Middle American household. My parents have to look in a mirror to know they are black. My mother still gets her hair straightened!" Michele said, touching her own striking "natural."

SOUL FOOD WAS WRONG FOR MICHELE

Michele was heavily into soul food, "of course." But when she explored her relationship to food more deeply, she discovered that she really didn't like the taste, especially the aftertaste, of much of that food. She ate hominy grits and chitterlings and pigs' knuckles because they seemed to be part of her black identity, which she wanted to emphasize, not because those foods provided her with a pleasurable eating experience.

Michele rarely enjoyed her meals. She processed food, eating very quickly. She also ate large quantities to prove to herself that she was really eating this food.

What turned out to hum for Michele were mostly "Middle American" foods, many of them plain, conventional dishes. Only after she could accept that tuna casserole and cherry pie were no threats to her blackness could she find pleasure in eating. She started to eat a wider range of foods, and only as much as she really felt like. After she tuned into her body signals in this way, she began to lose weight (or, to be more precise, her weight "got lost") as she was freed from the tyranny of food.

The idea that you should eat certain foods because most people in your family or group or commune eat them is deeply ingrained in society. Many times this is true to such an extent that people are unaware of this restricting influence.

Check yourself out on a few of these questions. Some are fairly universal, some apply only to certain cultural groups.

Select the ones that apply to you:

*   Can you imagine a big Sunday picnic without potato salad?
*   Before Thanksgiving Day, do you devote any time to finding out what main course you would really like?
*   Do you bake Christmas cookies in August?
*   Do you eat *latkes* (potato pancakes) in spring?
*   Have you ever eaten a mixed green salad for breakfast?
*   Have you ever had a sit-down fancy dinner party on the Fourth of July?
*   Do you ever make pumpkin pie in June?
*   Would you serve eggnog on Memorial Day?
*   Do you ever eat dessert before the main course?
*   Do you ever eat mustard greens for breakfast?

- Can you visualize having hamburgers and French fries for Easter dinner?
- Do you ever invite friends over after dinner for dessert and coffee?
- In a restaurant, would you ever order a bottle of Burgundy or other red wine with fish?
- Would you serve cranberry sauce with hamburgers?
- Have you tried split pea soup or minestrone or borscht for breakfast?
- Do you ever make gefilte fish on Monday?
- Do you ever put ice in your wine?
- Do you sometimes have fish for Sunday dinner?
- Would you ever serve blueberry muffins with lasagna?
- Do you ever eat hot cereal for dinner?

We have no intention of telling you that you *should* do any of these things. Some may seem bizarre, un-American, or quaint. But it is often helpful to become aware of how much of your eating is influenced and regulated by conventions and customs. And it is also worthwhile to be aware of your range of options, depending on your personal taste preferences.

Now, go over the list again, slowly, and try to visualize actually tasting or eating the items described at the times mentioned. Take a few moments with each one. Perhaps you can close your eyes as you visualize each one.

Do any combinations sound or feel intriguing, even tempting?

ARE YOU A CREATURE OF FOOD HABITS?

Jessica, the early-fiftyish mother of two sons in college, told our workshop that she had come to see that she was totally a creature of habit, and she felt this had been detrimental to her whole relationship to food.

"Everything is automatic. On Fridays, I automatically buy fish, even though the church has long since dropped the Friday no-meat rule. Sunday dinner is always at 2:30 p.m., and Sunday supper is always cold cuts, cheese, and salad. We've had ham every Easter of my life, and turkey with cornbread stuffing every Thanksgiving and Christmas. I feel like I'm in a four-foot rut!"

She felt that her eating had become as automatic as her shopping, cooking, and serving of food, and she was ready to change.

At Christmas when her sons came home from college, she tried to tune in to what hummed to her — and it definitely wasn't turkey! She felt rather courageous when she suggested to her husband and her sons that they all go to a restaurant for Christmas dinner, because she simply didn't feel like cooking a turkey.

To her total surprise, the three men assured her they really weren't that fond of turkey. But they also said they didn't want to go to a restaurant. Eating at home as a family unit was essential to their enjoyment of Christmas. Turkey was dispensable!

They finally compromised. Each of them would buy or prepare two or three favorite hors d'oeuvres for himself, with enough to share if others wanted some.

"We ended up with the most incredible buffet," Jessica reported. "I made cold sliced fillet of beef with Cumberland sauce and a tomato aspic with shrimp. One of the boys found a delicatessen that had the most marvelous *dolmas* and a very interesting Near Eastern millet salad. The other bought a can of Macadamia nuts and smoked oysters and little cocktail franks. And my husband, who never goes near the kitchen, made superb deviled eggs and sliced cucumbers in sour cream.

"It was the most exciting and yet relaxed Christmas dinner we've ever had. And we felt so close to each other, sharing an intimate event."

If you can feel free to reject food conventions and are aware of what you really want, then food is no longer tyrannizing you. Further, new sources of food pleasuring become available.

WHAT IF NOTHING HUMS?

What we frequently encounter, though, are people who tell us: "At last I know what I *don't* want, but I don't know what I *do* want."

There is no simple answer to that dilemma. Perhaps, incredible as it may be to consider, you really don't want anything at all, for now. So why not simply wait for your body's next signal?

Or, as we mentioned earlier, several things may be humming at once. Then it can be useful to ask yourself, "Would I feel cheated if I didn't have Number One? How about Number Two? Number Three?" You might even want some of each, and each would be humming loudly. Try some of each. There need be no more "death-row dinners"; you no longer have to feel guilty. And you are free to find food that pleasures and satisfies you; you have the freedom to choose.

The real long-range solution for the "multiple hummer" is heightened awareness. As with any knowledge of the self, such awareness grows gradually. Certain experiments and exercises can initiate this growth and promote it, but it is essentially an ongoing process.

We urge you not to be discouraged if at this point you still cannot always tell what is humming to you. Most people we have worked with have the same experience, even if they are really tuned into the liberated approach to eating. They also report, almost without exception, that the going gets easier and that after a while the signals start getting through loud and clear. Some report that food not only hums, it sings, or shouts!

Another aid in tuning in to these signals is coming up.

10/MANAGING THE FOOD-LIBERATED FAMILY AND CHILDREN

This chapter is for people who eat together as a family. It is about the traditional role of women (guardian of the kitchen, food preparer, and family nutritionist) and the traditional role of men as family chairman. We have unique suggestions to end family food hassles and help your children grow up without food hang-ups.

"I resent it when they don't eat what I've cooked. I feel like I've put myself on the table."
— Ella, forty-one, mother of two teenagers, 135 pounds

"The dinner table is like a tribunal. I eat as fast as I can and then get the hell out of there."
— Larry, sixteen, oldest of three boys, 208 pounds

"Dinner is the time for playing the *pater familias* role: Carve the meat, pour the wine, settle

squabbles, give everybody their share of attention, and show that you care about them."

— Gordon, forty-five, father of
three, 237 pounds

The family dinner's values, real or imagined, go far
beyond quenching thirst and stilling hunger. To many people
it has become the most tangible sign of cohesiveness of the
family unit. The prevailing philosophy is: Families who eat
together stay together, and are literally intact; members of
such a family feel they are retaining a sense of sharing and
keeping the channels of communication open.

"Eating dinner together as a family is as basic to American society as opening gifts together at Christmas" is the way
it was put by Eric, a thirty-five-year-old CPA and the father of
one young child. He continued, "And here you come along and
say it's O.K. for Mother to eat alone in her bedroom or to skip
Christmas dinner!"

We realize that the family dinner, as an institution, has
values. (The Pearson family enjoys many pleasurable meals
together.) But it's important that eating activities and social
ritual not become rigidly intertwined or confused. Could you
accept that one or more people in your family might not *feel*
like eating with the rest of you at times? Would that be O.K.?

In many families, dinnertime is the time for assuming
ritualized roles. For example, during one of our weekend
workshops Gordon realized that dinner was the time when he
assumed the stance of master (or chairman) of the household.
He felt he was expected to preside at the dinner table. He
assumed the tradition-assigned duties of the "provider" and

"breadwinner" — carve the turkey or the roast, dish out the meat, listen to a thumbnail account of everybody's day, settle arguments, be sure that the wife gets recognition via praise for her cooking, correct the children on their table manners, etc. And these are just the overt activities and verbal messages. On top of all this, he was supposed to taste, savor, and find pleasure in his food.

A housewife often expends much of her day's energies on activities related to dinner — shopping and cooking. She feels that her husband's and children's health are primarily her responsibility because she usually buys and prepares the food that nourishes them and also expects to please them esthetically. If her family doesn't enjoy the taste and appearance of the meal, or if someone eats too little or even rejects part of the meal, she can easily feel put down. She is getting poor marks as Mother, the custodian of health and well-being. She may even feel that all the time she spent planning and preparing the meal was wasted.

If the family does eat and fully appreciates the meal, Mother feels rewarded and recognized. However, she often has difficulty focusing on her *own* food enjoyment, what with her responsibilities for serving the family.

HOW FAMILY DINNERS CAN HURT CHILDREN

Children are most overtly the beneficiaries of the meal ritual. They are being cared for. Attention is being given to them. In many families, this is the prime time that both parents set aside for focusing on the children, letting them discuss their experiences of the day and sharing their successes and concerns. The child may bask in this attention. Or he may also feel, as Larry put it, that dinner is a tribunal, a time for being judged or put on the spot.

Also, children can be subjected to an incredible number of put-downs regarding food and their eating. If a child doesn't eat much, he may be told that he is endangering his future health. As if that isn't enough of a threat, the disadvantages of sickness are often irrelevantly pointed out, as in "Do you want to get sick and have to stay home when we go to the game Saturday?"

Further, the child is often made to feel guilty for being unappreciative: "All the time I spent fixing this meal for you — and all you do is sit and poke at it!" Eating or not eating becomes tied to approval, acceptance, love.

These particular scenes may not occur in your family, but there is a veritable arsenal of emotionally loaded issues that can hinder, if not prevent, eating pleasure at dinnertime.

We have found that in many families, conflicts and problems are aired principally at the dinner table. It's usually the first (and perhaps the only) time of day when the family comes together as a unit, and if problems are hanging in the air they often are served up right along with dinner.

In other families everyone is in a rush to eat and get on with something else. The mood is hectic. Maybe everybody is talking, but there is very little listening or relating to one another.

The range of patterns of family relationships at dinnertime is almost infinite. Our point is: *Explore effective times and places for your family to share and be together, other than at the dinner table every night.* In today's super-busy atmosphere this may be difficult, but we believe that the separation of food enjoyment from extraneous emotions will help every member of the family — and not just in managing their weight.

We have found that it is possible to provide a family with greater eating freedom without creating anarchy in the kitchen or dining room. This requires clear rules and understandings worked out together by all the family members.

Freedom to eat what you like, when you like it, does not mean an end to sharing and being together. Most families find that they actually do eat many meals together under our system, and they often eat the same foods. However, knowing that they don't *have to*, that they can skip a meal when they're not hungry — knowing they can choose different foods without hurting anybody's feelings — makes all this a matter of choice, rather than obligation. This feeling of freedom and choice puts fun back into family meals and times together.

In the Pearson household, the family often gets together after dinner in the living room for an hour of talk or cards or Monopoly or other games with the children. We often find this time preferable to using the dinner ritual for being together.

What are the possibilities, what can happen, if you accept the validity of being together but not necessarily eating together?

Everyone can fix his own meal and eat alone or sit with whomever he prefers.

• The housewife prepares a dinner, selecting foods that *she* likes — or that one member requested — and if that food doesn't hum to another family member, he can fix something else or eat later, if that is what he feels like.

• Mother serves dinner to very young children to suit their preferences and schedule; the adults recognize that they have different tastes and therefore eat at a different time and different foods, but still everybody spends some time together later.

• The family may eat dinner separately, but may enjoy dessert together.

• The family has a communal dinner. Everyone prepares what hums to him. If the children are old enough to fix food themselves, a family potluck can be fun.

COMPROMISE EATING WHERE NO ONE WINS

Marilyn and Peter were one couple with a family dinner problem. She was of Russian background; his family was part Hungarian and part Italian. Peter was fond of rice and pasta; Marilyn found that potatoes really hummed to her. Marilyn enjoyed soups; Peter didn't. Marilyn loved sweet gelatin salads; Peter yearned for tossed green salads or coleslaw. Marilyn was fascinated with a variety of exotic foods; Peter preferred to stick to familiar tastes.

Over the years they had worked out what they considered a good compromise between their tastes. However, they came to realize the compromise satisfied neither. Marilyn very often cooked meals that had little appeal to her, although the food might beckon once it was on the table. She thought it her duty to prepare dishes Peter liked and she rarely bothered to fix something else just for herself.

Peter, at the same time, often found food on the table that held no gustatory attraction for him. But he ate it as a matter of courtesy to his wife: "It's always tasty and carefully prepared — it's just that it often wasn't humming to me."

Their eating compromise reminded us of the famous O. Henry story "The Gift of the Magi," in which both husband and wife make a severe sacrifice of something treasured, only to find that their gifts and their sacrifices have cancelled each other out. (She sold her beautiful long hair to buy him a watch chain; he sold his treasured watch to buy her an elegant hair comb.)

Marilyn and Peter's compromise had worked so both of them were out of touch with food enjoyment. Consequently, both became overeaters and acquired weight problems.

Is anything comparable happening in your family?

Recall your last meal together as a family. Concentrate now on several different aspects of the meal.

HOW ABOUT THE FOOD?

Did you enjoy it? Are you fully aware of what you ate? Try to remember every single dish you had for dinner last night. If you cannot remember each item clearly, if some dishes made no definite impression, do you think it is because you were too distracted from the eating experience? Or do you think the reason lies with the food, that it was unimaginative or prosaic and therefore made no impact? Did you have a feeling of wanting something else when dinner was over?

HOW ABOUT THE SOCIAL PART OF DINNER?

Did you enjoy being with the people who were at the table? Did their presence mean something to you? Could you give them your undivided attention when they spoke? Did they give you the attention you felt you deserved? When it was over, what was your mood?

HOW ABOUT THE MEAL'S TOTAL EMOTIONAL VALUE?

What kind of feeling do you have about the whole experience? Warm and tender? Indifferent? Do you value the sharing of the meal? Or do you feel slightly deprived of food sensations? Do your eating partners enjoy you and vice versa? Or do you feel put down in any way by them? In retrospect, was this one of the better parts of your day? Or were you glad when it was over? Did you dread it in any way prior to sitting down? Do you solve so many problems at the dinner table or share feelings so intensely that you cannot focus on your food?

Once they stop to examine the complex fabric of the family dinner, some people find themselves with ambiguous and even conflicting feelings about its values as a daily ritual.

Often, eating together as a family is similar to watching TV or reading a book while eating: you're so engrossed in the events, the people, or the plot that the food is hardly tasted.

Again, we suggest that you might find it helpful to keep a journal or diary. Keep track of the degree of satisfaction you get from your meals in terms of specific foods, times, places, settings, people. Once a week or every two weeks review your field notes, almost like an anthropologist studying the eating patterns of a culture and tribe. Determine which occasions were most pleasurable, which were frustrating or uncomfortable. See what you can learn about situations that could be enhanced, others that could be avoided.

As you become clearer within yourself, can you discuss this entire matter with the people you eat with (though preferably not at dinnertime)? Husband and wife might have a discussion between themselves first. But children, unless they are very young, should be brought into the conference, too. About the only ground rules you need is to ask everyone to be honest, because you're trying to work out a plan that will satisfy everyone.

WANTED: MORE RELAXATION

Gordon found in his family he wasn't the only one who was uncomfortable about his role. His wife and children all expressed themselves clearly: They wanted a more relaxed and informal atmosphere. They had not wanted to offend him by raising the issue before this time. For this particular family, more relaxed eating included these points:

Dinner didn't always have to be exactly at 6:00 P.M. If there was a special TV program, or if Nancy (Gordon's wife) had been busy in the afternoon, or if he had had a rough day and wanted a shower before dinner, the meal hour could be moved up or back.

It wasn't an insult to the rest of the family if one or another family member stayed away from the dinner table because he wanted to eat earlier, or later, or by himself, or *not to eat at all*.

Dinner no longer had to consist of the traditional salad, a main course of meat, vegetables, and a starchy food, and then dessert. Sometimes they only had two kinds of medium-sized pizza, or soup and dessert. And once in a while dinner consisted of only desserts!

Prior to dinner, the children were allowed to join in the cocktail hour with a soft drink or fruit juice in the living room. *This became the time and place for Dad to settle squabbles and find out what was going on at home and at school.* Soon the dinner conversation became more relaxed and free of pressure to resolve disputes.

Another family tried alternate times for togetherness. On days when they did not eat together, they usually gathered in the living room around 8:00 P.M. for "party" time. This often included a time-limited game of Monopoly or dominoes, checkers, etc. The kids loved these occasions because they found they could then count on the genuine attention of both parents.

This time together could also mean sitting by the fire and sipping hot apple cider on cold nights; it could mean the family's watching a favorite TV program together and then discussing it, it could even be the quiet sharing of everybody finding the most comfortable place to sit or lie with a book. The same family also instituted frequent menu planning sessions, when every member of the family had a chance to make requests and register objections.

Another way to achieve togetherness, which this family had never attempted previously, was joint shopping expeditions, or as one West Coast preteener put it, "Safeway safaris." This ties in closely with something we find essential in our own family: Keeping an open shopping list, a sheet of paper or pad in an accessible place, where everyone can write down food requests. (We keep ours on a magnetic pad on the refrigerator door.)

This enables every family member to state his likes. If a request cannot be met, it is still not ignored. If somebody asks for filet mignon every night and the family budget is more attuned to casseroles and hamburgers, this can be discussed.

CHILDREN REACT SENSIBLY

Most parents are amazed at how few, if any, unreasonable demands their children make when they are assured they do have a voice in the family food management.

"I was afraid they would ask for all thirty-one varieties of Baskin-Robbins's ice cream," said Mary, the mother of five. "Instead, all they want is to be sure there is always chocolate, strawberry, and butterscotch topping in the house."

Marilyn and Peter made a significant change in their relationship to food and to each other: Marilyn now rarely cooks those of Peter's favorites that she dislikes. He sometimes cooks them himself; more often he eats them at a restaurant or brings them home from a place that has his humming food "to go."

He sometimes calls her from work late in the afternoon and tells her what's humming to him. If it appeals to her and it's feasible to do, she prepares it. If it doesn't, or if it's inconvenient, he gets it himself. When she does serve his kind of food, she feels free to make something else for herself.

Peter and Marilyn found that *this freer relationship has carried over into aspects of their lives that are not related to food.* They have relaxed their attitude toward household chores, which they had previously handled on a strict basis of man's work versus woman's work versus children's work.

They initially doubted that their children would benefit from greater food freedom, but decided to give it a try because "the kids couldn't become worse eaters than they are now." They were more than mildly surprised to find that the children *did* eat more when allowed to choose for themselves, and that they ate very little "junk stuff," provided they knew it was in the house and available whenever they wanted.

Peter and Marilyn had worried about their children being skinny and not eating well. Most obese parents have the opposite worry: They have a deep, overriding fear that their obesity, like a family curse, will be handed down from generation to generation.

Cynthia, a thirty-three-year-old part-time bookkeeper who was nearly forty pounds overweight, lived with this gnawing fear. She argued that her mother had been fat, her grandmother had been fat, she was fat, and so undoubtedly her only daughter, Sharon, would have to be fat, too. She watched every bite Sharon put in her mouth, admonishing her to stay away from the starchy, high-calorie "junk" and at the same time lecturing her on the need for sufficient protein, vitamins, and minerals, and the right balance of nutrients.

At age eight, Sharon could have taught Adele Davis a thing or two about nutrition. She was also decidedly chubby.

Cynthia, a graduate of several weight-watching organizations, found it extremely difficult to look upon food as a source of pleasure. At first she flatly said she could not teach such a doctrine to Sharon: "It would be a complete about-face. I have always taught her about nutrition and health as the guiding factors in eating."

Cynthia attributed Sharon's overweight to her daughter's sweet tooth: "I know that whenever I'm not looking she gets ice cream and candy." Cynthia herself ate sweets whenever she broke out of dietary prison.

After several weeks during which Cynthia got more in touch with her own way of using food and the fact that sweets were necessary pleasure foods for her at times, she took the plunge. When she discussed it, she couldn't hold back the tears.

She took Sharon to a candy store and told her that she could pick out a one-pound box with any combination of candies and chocolates she wanted. The child was incredulous, and finally asked what the special occasion was. "Nothing special," Cynthia said. "I just think it's time you and I shared some of our favorite foods. I'm buying a pound box for myself, and the one you chose will be all yours."

At this, the little girl threw her arms around her mother and blurted out, with tears in her eyes, "Oh Mommy, I didn't know you loved me that much."

After this episode Cynthia gave Sharon much more food freedom and tried not to weigh the nutritional value of every bite the child ate. In the past she had also kept her daughter out of the kitchen, the place of temptation. Now she allowed Sharon to join her in preparing dishes and started to introduce her to simple projects like preparing instant pudding and baking brownies from a mix.

Sharon loved cooking, and loved sharing adult activities with her mother. "We have so much mutual fun now with our old enemy, food," her mother reported on one of our Institute follow-up questionnaires. "And we have lost twenty pounds between us — me sixteen and Sharon four."

With a very young child, naturally, parents need to make a preselection. Also, mothers of young children have enough work without becoming short-order cooks and preparing different foods for every member of the family. Do only what is comfortable and convenient. Gradually introduce changes as you have time and energy. For example, some choice can be offered even to a very young child without straining Mother's energies or the family budget. From the standpoint of nutrition and mother's time and budget, it makes little difference whether a child eats his tomatoes sliced or whole; whether he gets chunky or smooth peanut butter, or raisin or chocolate-chip cookies.

WHY SMALL CHOICES MAKE BIG DIFFERENCES

But all these very small choices can make a big difference to the young child. Being consulted about them, being able to make decisions on these simple but important matters, gives him a good, free feeling about his eating: *He isn't eating for Mommy or Daddy*; he is eating for himself. And he is learning to make choices and exercise options.

The attitude that he should eat to please someone other than himself is one of the most destructive that can be implanted in a child. Think about it: "A spoonful for Mommy; a spoonful for Daddy; a spoonful for Auntie Jane; a spoonful for the nice man who brings our mail" — over the years, if not centuries, these coaxings undoubtedly have produced legions of mixed-up eaters and overweight adults.

It is quite true that overweight parents tend to have overweight children, but only a small percentage of this is due to heredity, in the physical sense. It happens mostly because parents communicate their feelings and attitudes about food to their children.

For example, Marcia, a twenty-seven-year-old divorcee with a weight problem of over fifty pounds, centered much of her life on her only child, six-year-old Lisa. To Marcia's horror, Lisa had also become overweight. And despite the mother's hawk-like surveillance of the child, the problem seemed to be escalating with every monthly checkup.

We explored with Marcia her daughter's eating problem as well as her own. Incredibly, Lisa's food passion was fruit yoghurt. But her mother and the grandmother, who baby-sat with her after kindergarten, worried that by eating too much yoghurt the child would not get proper nutrition.

Many parents religiously follow nutritional and calorie charts in deciding what their children should eat daily. In this case, the two women were in constant battle with Lisa, keeping yoghurt from her and trying to make her eat a perfectly "balanced" health-chart diet of milk, eggs, yellow and green vegetables, fruit, bread, and meat.

We suggested to this family that the child be allowed her beloved yoghurt, but that mother and grandmother continue to *offer* her a variety of foods and tell her of their value without pressuring her. Also, if she thought it was indicated, we suggested that Marcia consider giving her daughter multivitamins until her diet stabilizes with a reasonable variety of foods.

However, this was one family we failed to help. The grandmother, who prepared most of Lisa's meals, wasn't able to relinquish her role as guardian of health and nutrition. Perhaps it helped her feel more needed. At any rate, Marcia felt powerless to change her mother's ideas about children's nutritional needs and eating patterns, and she wasn't prepared to do all-out battle.

We have known other mothers whose wish to spare their children the curse of obesity caused them to resort to various maneuvers. They may offer high-calorie food to a child, but grimace or in some other way try to get across the message "This is bad." Some of these mothers make a show of hating things like cake and candy and loving celery sticks or low-fat cottage cheese.

A mother who resorts to this trickery is doing herself and her child a serious disservice. Children are highly attuned to picking up nonverbal messages, so they aren't easily deceived, so the mother has mostly undermined her own position. At the same time, she is teaching the child to ignore body signals in relation to food.

NEVER MIND THE SPINACH

We believe that the first step toward establishing a free relationship to food and liberated eating is for a child to realize that his parents derive genuine pleasure from their own eating and want him to experience similar pleasure. This means letting the child reject foods he cannot abide and enjoy foods he prefers.

The "Popeye syndrome" has been the bane of existence of several generations of American youngsters. We have yet to hear any plausible explanation why a child who doesn't like spinach (and few do) cannot get the same vitamins and other nutrients from other green vegetables and fruits.

Letting a child pleasure himself with food entails several other changes. One is the need to offer variety. Another is to allow the child to express natural curiosity and to experiment with (and explore) foods.

Parents sometimes think they are providing their child with a variety of taste experiences by insisting that the child "try just one bite" of every food on the table. This compulsory exploring often backfires. If the child resents having to try, the concept of exploration becomes contaminated; a child may end up unwilling to sample anything unfamiliar.

Parents who explore new foods themselves create a model for their children. If there is no coercion, the child's inherent curiosity will take over. Modern education places much emphasis on exploration and experimentation to develop "self-directed learners." To become a self-directed eater, a child must be allowed experimentation.

This does mean forgetting about "manners" — at least sometimes. Many of the steps we go through in food-awareness exercises come naturally to a child: He wants to touch the inside of foods, like a banana or an apricot; he wants to lick potato chips and other foods; he wants to stir his ice-cream till it's almost soft enough to drink; he wants to nibble on crackers or cookies "like a bunny rabbit," using just his front teeth; he wants to try how mayonnaise would taste on a poached egg.

Most of the time, his trips of discovery are cut short with "Stop that, that's not polite." Or "Will you try to eat like a human being?" Or "That's a childish way to eat!"

Letting your child experiment at times (it needn't be when Grandma is over for her birthday dinner) will help him to know what food is all about and to grow up without some of the hang-ups many of us have to tackle as adults.

One family noticed on their first camping trip with their children, aged two and four, how tranquil meals had suddenly become. They came to realize that this happier mood came about because they were allowing the children more freedom with their food and didn't worry too much about manners. At home, the constant preoccupation with

"Finish your plate" and "Don't spill it on the floor" and "Your face is dirty" had made mealtimes extremely tense and unrewarding for everybody.

The major concern about children's eating that we hear from parents is "What about sweets? Where do you set the limits there? I couldn't just let them eat all they want!"

Several studies have shown that a young child, if given a range of choices of various foods, will in time balance his own diet. We mentioned one such study by Dr. Margaret Ribble a few chapters back. Another one, by Dr. Clara Davis, is reported at length in a book that most families have on their own bookshelf, Dr. Benjamin Spock's *Baby and Child Care.*

This is of little comfort to a mother who sees that despite all her admonitions, her child is eating far too many sweets. To be practical, most parents will realize that their child will probably eat candy no matter what they do. The fact that sweets are forbidden often makes them even more desirable. At any rate, the child who really wants sweets will sneak them if they are withheld. He may trade with classmates or may use his lunch money for chocolate.

We have these suggestions:
If you are concerned over your child's imbalanced diet, give him vitamin pills. This will at least partially relieve your worries.

•   Provide him with high-quality candies. We do not mean substitutes or low-calorie candies, but chocolate and candy of good quality, and especially cakes, cookies, and pies made with excellent ingredients. Whenever possible, teach him that only the best is worth eating.

157

- It is often practical to give each child in a family a "goodie" allowance — a fixed amount of money to be used totally at that person's discretion. This must not be mixed up with a child's general allowance or be used for family treats, such as desserts for everyone. This is money the individual may spend, personally or via entries on the family shopping list, entirely at his own discretion and totally for *himself* regardless of what food it is.

If a teen-age daughter puts pecan or Boston cream pie on the shopping list as her special goodie, this doesn't mean "we'll all have pecan pie for dessert tonight." It should mean only that she has pecan pie to eat whenever she wants.

At the same time, parents should refrain from bringing children treats that haven't been requested.

HOW TO MAKE CANDY LAST FOR WEEKS

Have you ever brought home a box of cookies and with-in minutes the family has demolished the entire box? Usually this happens because everyone feels they have to eat fast to get their fair share. So everyone digs in, whether it's humming or not. Most families who have tried letting their children have their own package of cookies or box of candy find that it lasts a remarkably long time.

Since food is one of life's basic pleasures and is also a basic security, mothers frequently are amazed to report that a box of candy not only lasts several weeks but even remains unopened for quite a while. Obviously, the key is for the child to *know it is there and available* if and when he wants it.

Family treats are an entirely different matter. Once every few months, the Pearson family has all-dessert dinner. Everybody puts in his request for a favorite cake or pie (or prepares it) and then the family dines on this buffet of sweets. The first course might be cherry pie a la mode. Second course: four kinds of cookies. Third course: ice-cream cake, etc.

This kind of unorthodox eating has worked well for many families. Of course, each family has to make up its own rules, based on individual needs and financial limitations.

DIETING PARENTS CAN CREATE OBESE CHILDREN

John and Ellen and their two children are an example of one family that worked out a unique system because of new insights. Both parents were thirty-five. Ellen said she had never gotten back her figure after Brian, now twelve, was born, and had put on more weight after the birth of Tracy, now seven. She was about twenty pounds "over." John, an attorney, was almost forty pounds overweight and reported that he had "always had a weight problem. I've practically been weaned on skim milk because I was too heavy and my mother had me on a diet since I was three or four, no pastries — the whole trip."

Their children were described to us as overweight, "finicky eaters who only like junk food that's not healthy for them."

During eating exercises and food fantasies, Ellen and John found that practically everything that hummed to them were foods they had not eaten in years, such as cream pies and French bread with sweet butter.

Ellen had geared her menus entirely to "the kind of nutritious foods that are good for children. I didn't want them turning out like us!" Her own and her husband's likes were given hardly any consideration. Nor, for that matter, were the children's. They were being fed what Mother considered healthful for them. The point was never made that a food could be delicious or exciting. The basic question was: How nutritious is it?

It was difficult for these parents to rethink their own relationship to food and to allow such criteria as enjoyment and pleasure to become primary. But both were convinced that there had been something decidedly wrong with the old eating style, since they saw the very results they dreaded and were trying to avoid — fat children — before their eyes. They decided to experiment.

One experiment involved taking the whole family to a restaurant that featured a fine, extensive smorgasbord. The children were told they could eat whatever and however much they wanted. Brian loaded up his plate, but ate only about half before saying, "Wow, I give up! Can I get cake even if I leave this?" He was assured that he could; he got his cake, ate, and declared, "I am full, I couldn't eat another bite."

Tracy took nibbles of almost everything and had a great time exploring the many different dishes, commenting on how soft or sour or chewy (or whatever) they were. She picked chocolate chiffon pie for her dessert, but left the crust.

What struck John and Ellen was that both children had not eaten particularly large amounts and that both of them ate a variety, some of it "good, healthy stuff — meats and salads, very little bread. They took plenty of sweet stuff, but they didn't finish it!"

After this experience, Ellen instituted the open shopping list in her kitchen. She also made what turned out to be a critical change: She stopped serving food portioned out on individual plates. Instead, she served it in dishes from which everybody would help himself. If there were any leftovers from the night before, she warmed them up and put them on the table, so that there was often more choice.

At least once every two weeks, the family made up its own smorgasbord, and everyone was allowed to name one or two dishes — "one if it's complicated or expensive; two if they're simple." Everybody also joined in the preparation, with Brian and Tracy usually doing gelatin salads and deviled eggs and John cooking up a big pot of chili.

After a few months, the children had stabilized their weight and both parents had started to lose weight, without trying to. Most important, the family's daily battleground had become a new occasion for enjoyment and togetherness. "Mealtime," said Ellen, "used to be all nagging and scolding and worrying. Now it's fun."

Of course, different families need to explore different alternatives. In the majority of cases we have dealt with, the relaxing of rules and offering greater choice were important.

Liberation is often the key to beginning the process of problem solving, especially the liberation of children from such dicta as "Stop being so fussy"; "We all have to eat some things we don't like"; "Eat it, it's good for you"; "Your grandmother worked hard to cook this for you — don't disappoint her"; "There are children in India, Africa, and China who would be happy to have this meal"; "You won't grow up strong and healthy if you don't eat better than that"; "When I was your age, I ate twice that"; "Don't play with your food"; "No dessert for you, if that's all you're going to eat"; "Finish your plate, dear"; "As soon as you finish your meat, I'll get you some ice cream"; "Just *taste* some of it."

Summing up, here are some ideas we have found helpful in the parent-child-food relationship:

- Giving children an opportunity to learn about foods and explore foods.
- Providing them with variety and choice.
- Not turning them *off* food by too many admonitions about nutritional value.
- Allowing them to select and eat what they enjoy.
- Allowing them to reject what they don't like.
- Not interfering with their personal style of eating.
- Giving them a voice in the family food selection.
- Letting them have their own box of candy or bag of cookies.
- Giving them a goodie allowance.
- Letting them fix meals for themselves as soon as they are able to (with most children, this is possible by the time they are nine or ten).
- Letting them observe parents pleasuring themselves with food.

- Not tying eating to emotions such as love and appreciation.

- Respecting the child's individuality and his preferences.

- Not allowing food to become a battlefield between parent and child. This is a battle that both lose.

- Being aware of the subtle events that happen at your dinner table. For example, you don't need to offer each other food that's visible and available on the table. People can ask for it. "Would you like some . . . ? ," is usually a seduction or an unnecessary invitation to foods that beckon but don't hum.

Part II

EXERCISES

FOR FOOD AND DRINK AWARENESS

AND SENSUOUS EATING

11/ *TEST YOUR FOOD FEELINGS HERE*

"What do you like best in the world, Pooh?"

"Well," said Pooh, "what I like best —" and then he had to stop and think.

Because although Eating Honey *was* a very good thing to do, there was a moment just before you began to eat it which was better than when you were, but he didn't know what it was called.

—A. A. Milne
The House at Pooh Corner

People trying to understand their own psychology of eating may share Pooh's experience. Often it is disappointing to find that a food you craved doesn't come up to expectations when you taste it.

The relationship between a person and food is never static. "I like coconut-almond-fudge ice cream" is a correct statement for only right now, for this precise moment. It's possible that a specific flavor of ice cream hums to you more often than anything else. It may be the central theme in your personal symphony of foods. But it is important to keep yourself open to the almost infinite number of variations you are capable of enjoying.

Once in a while people take their first steps toward awareness — getting in touch with their likes and dislikes — and then regress. They put themselves in a box and insist rigidly: "I don't want food between meals"; "I am an original breadoholic."

This is definitely a better place to be than being regulated by someone else's dictum, such as "You must have a high-protein food for breakfast." At least you started from something uniquely yours when you classified yourself as a bread freak.

We are saying that you need to stay aware of the possibility of change — in fact, the likelihood of shifts and swings in eating preferences. You cannot tune in to your needs once; *tuning in is a continuing process.*

To open up to this process it is essential to view every moment as "now," to stay in the *now*, in the present awareness, rather than calculate and computerize along such lines as: "I haven't eaten since this morning, and it's mealtime." "I'm losing weight and should be hungry because of all that fat I've burned off." "I wanted pasta last week and just couldn't get it." "I am not going to have time to eat until much later today, so I'd better eat more and store up against hunger."

Instead, ask yourself this question: " *What do I feel like eating or drinking right now, if anything?*" If you are confused whether something is humming or only beckoning, we again suggest that you ask: "*Will I feel cheated if I don't have it now?*"

The main idea is to check out what you want on the basis of your present feelings, not your "track record" from the past or expectations of the future, and not on when you last ate or might be able to eat again later.

One workshop participant felt frightened because for almost two days during the weekend she had felt absolutely no hunger and hadn't eaten anything. She wondered, "How much longer can this go on? Surely, I *must* be hungry!" But she wasn't — not until Sunday afternoon. This woman had never before closely examined whether she was hungry before she ate, let alone considered what precise food she was hungry for.

Sometimes staying in the "now" is difficult because a person is concerned about whether foods are going to be available when wanted. In workshops, people have described fantasies or nightmares about Eskimo Ice Cream, or Barton's Chocolates, or Pepsi-Cola, or other companies going out of business or discontinuing a specific item; or of stores in their city no longer stocking a favorite brand; or of a strike that would stop all deliveries of a favorite food or beverage.

Most of these "endangered species" of foods are not perishable. (We have never met anyone who worried that cottage cheese or spinach would vanish.) Generally, the worrisome food is a particular kind of candy bar, a specific canned (and sometimes frozen) food. It is possible and sensible to lay in a good supply of these and keep restocking long before the supply is gone.

Staying in the "now," and responding to your needs and cravings as they develop, can sometimes lead to unexpected explorations and adventures in eating. For example, Roxanne, a thirty-nine-year-old department-store executive, described at an advanced workshop what she called a roller-coaster ride:

"I was scared — I craved sausage pizzas almost every day, practically from the time I opened my eyes. That food had been a no-no for eight years, and I forbade myself to eat it. As I said, craving it so constantly after the basic workshop [six weeks earlier] scared me, but I was determined to go with my humming. I didn't eat an awful lot. I guess that was partly because I knew there were more pizzas waiting, and partly because I had really given myself permission to eat what I wanted. After five or six days, pizza lost its appeal.

"Suddenly, I became excited about Mexican food — *chili rellenos*, refried beans, tacos, enchiladas, guacamole, tostados — all of it! Another world of illicit food that I managed to avoid for years. I followed my hum: Mexican dinner every night! This lasted about a week.

"After that I went on a Chinese-food kick — lots of wonton soup, sweet-sour pork, egg rolls, fried shrimp with that super-hot mustard, mandarin chicken, chow mein, pea pods with water chestnuts, the works. That was fun. I forget exactly how long that lasted. About ten days. I know it sounds crazy, but next I developed a craving for cauliflower and other hard vegetables. I'm still exploring that world now!"

To stay in touch with yourself in the present, it is also important to be aware of your current emotions and moods. They play an important role in harmonious eating. We have developed an exercise to assist in this process, the Food-Awareness Test which follows. As we mentioned earlier, food awareness is not a static condition but a process. It keeps growing and developing. Therefore, this test is something you might want to repeat periodically, even after you have finished this book.

BEFORE YOU TAKE THE FOOD-AWARENESS TEST

This is a pencil-and-paper exercise designed to provide you with more information about yourself and the emotional uses you make of food. Answer the questions spontaneously, without considering what would be the "best" answer, since there are no right or wrong answers! No one is going to score your paper.

We suggest that you keep it for your own future reference. Give yourself the same test again in a few weeks, and again in a few months; it would be interesting and informative to compare the results.

The test is presented on the next few pages, and space is provided so you can work directly in this book. If you got the book from a library or a friend or would rather not write in your copy, just get some plain paper and organize it exactly the way the next few pages are.

The test will present situations often associated with food, eating and drinking. These situations will reflect moods or emotions or relate to family members. Then you will be asked to associate a food or drink with that situation. Finally, you will be asked to describe the style or manner of eating or drinking that goes with that food.

For some situations, it's possible that no food or beverage will occur to you. That's all right. If nothing comes to mind after a few minutes, leave it blank. You can go back and review all your responses later.

There is no time limit — take all the time you need to respond to each item as best you can.

Reply to each item with whatever food or beverage comes to mind. Just write it down without any censoring.

For the "style of eating," use words like "fast" or "stand-up" or "feeling dumb" or "nibbling" or anything that fits the occasion.

After you have finished the list, take a few minutes for review. Try to fill in any blank spots, if at all possible. You may find that you have never associated some situations with food or eating. If so, watch these situations in the future and see what you in fact do and/or eat at those times. People often are surprised at how little aware they were of the foods and styles of eating connected with moods or associated with family.

Make any changes you wish. But do this only if something else feels more precise, not because you think it is more appropriate.

Now study the whole picture. What do you notice? Any puzzling or surprising discoveries? Any unusual links or clusters? Look over any foods that keep recurring. What do you observe about your use of certain foods in association with certain situations? Mark up your paper with connecting lines or arrows or underlines.

The Food-Awareness Test

(Complete each item before going on to the next one.)

Situation or mood	Food or drink	Style or manner of eating or drinking
1. Bored		
2. Fearful, afraid		
3. Fatigue		
4. Sad		
5. Depressed		
6. Angry		
7. Lonely		
8. Nervous or tense		
9. Self-hate or disgust		
10. Guilty		

Stop here for a few moments and look over your answers. Fill in any that you weren't able to do earlier, if possible. Now on to the next section.

Situation or mood	Food or drink	Style or manner of eating or drinking
11. Excited, delighted		
12. Sharing, companionship		
13. Playful, having fun		
14. Being alone (but not lonely)		
15. Luxuriousness		
16. Happy, joyful		

Stop here for a few moments. These have all been positive moods and see if there are any more blanks here. Can you fill any of them in? Now go on to the last section.

Situation	Food or drink	Style or manner of eating or drinking
17. Home (your own)		
18. Watching TV or reading		
19. Remembering mother		
20. Remembering father		
21. Remembering grandparents		
22. Childhood (your own)		
23. Being with mother (now)		
24. Being with father (now)		
25. Being with grandparents (now)		

To give a few examples (for illustration only, since everyone's responses will differ), your list might look something like this:

Situation / mood	Food or drink	Style or manner of eating or drinking
Fatigue	Tea with honey	Feet up; sipping
Boredom	Snacks, beer	Not very aware
Excitement, de-light	Usually nothing; maybe wine or snack foods	Nibbling; sipping
Worry	Dark milk choco-late	Licking; Gum-ming

The purposes of this exercise are:

(1) To help you become more aware of how you use food in response to emotions, situations, people.

(2) To help you in the future to identify your mood more clearly by your behavior. No one can be aware of his feelings all the time. For example, when you start to consume milk chocolate heavily, this can be a mood clue. In other words, food and your mode of eating can provide you with signals about your underlying emotional state.

(3) To enable you to be more efficient in satisfying yourself, whether through food or some other body comfort. For

instance, when you are bored, is there a particular style of eating that could enhance the effectiveness of the beer and/or snacks? Are there foods other than beer and snacks that might be more exciting and more likely to relieve your boredom and monotony?

(4) To make you aware of any specific food links to your past — childhood, mother, father, grandparents. Such knowledge is important in relating to food, and can be enhanced and built on further.

To some of our workshop members this has been strikingly important. One housewife, the mother of four children, realized that the foods that hummed to her in situations of worry, sadness, loneliness, nervousness and guilt, were all comfort foods she associated with her grandparents. As a child she deeply loved her grandparents, a kindly Austrian couple who owned a bakery, but her parents frequently quarreled with the grandparents and she often felt caught in the middle. As an adult, her feeling toward food was mostly one of guilt.

In her early life, the foods she associated with tenderness and love — pastries — were offered by her grandparents and forbidden by her parents. They often became a source of bitter quarrels among the adults. In later years, these foods were forbidden by all the parent-surrogate diets. After becoming aware of these associations, she could trace the layers of guilt wedged into each cream-puff. These comfort foods had never been allowed to do their "work."

A GUILT-BEGETS-GUILT CYCLE

Another workshop participant was startled as she realized what a vicious cycle she was caught in. Whenever she felt a negative emotion such as fear or sadness or anxiety, she turned to sweet and creamy foods. That would have been fine if she hadn't also felt guilty about eating such high-calorie foods. Then she would *relieve her guilt with sweet and creamy foods*, which kept her in an almost hopeless bind. She ate through a filter of guilt and ambivalence.

The key for her was to realize the legitimacy of using these creamy, sweet reward foods when she felt anxious or sad, and consequently not feel guilty about eating them. This broke the vicious cycle and also resulted in less food consumption and weight.

Many people find that the Food-Awareness Test helps them realize to what degree food and eating are a rich and valid part of their life. This is usually felt as a relief after the long period of alienation most overweight people have suffered through.

Most of the diet apostles and establishment nutritionists do their best to foster an unnatural and unhappy state of alienation. In their view, the proper perspective is not "person and food," but "person vs. food." For example, Jean Nidetch, the founder of Weight Watchers, in her book *Weight Watchers* (W/W Twentyfirst Corporation, 1970) expounds: "I enjoyed convincing people of their own power over themselves." There is no mention of power and wisdom *within* yourself, only of power *over* yourself — power to be marshaled and used against those arch enemies, food and overeating, in a pro-longed state of guerrilla warfare.

Weight Watchers also stresses that "food is for nutri-tion, not pleasure." This is a denial of all psychological knowl-edge about the emotional satisfactions in food and eating.

Another national dieters' group, Overeaters Anony-mous, passes out cards warning: "Abstinence is the most im-portant thing in my life without exception!" "Life Line," a pamphlet published by the same organization, contains the following "confession," delivered at a conference by a member who, presumably, accepted the group's philosophy that "com-pulsive overeating is a progressive illness. . . ." Previously, "I was united with food. What held me there? Ignorance, self -will and desire for immediate pleasure." *Disgusting* and *weak-willed* are the implied self-accusations.

The list could go on for pages, but most overweight people are all too familiar with this fight-the-enemy-food, fight-against-yourself approach.

What this warfare produces, along with weight prob-lems, alienation, deprivation, guilt, and staying out of touch with body wisdom, is something amply illustrated in all the "before" and "after" pictures these groups are fond of publish-ing: Thinking of yourself as a Thin Person or a Fat Person, not simply as a Person. (The "after-the-after" pictures are not published because diet programs are notoriously ineffective for long-range weight loss.)

Quite a few people, when we first encounter them, tell us that they have a fat personality and a thin personality, the thin one vastly superior to the fat one. The thin one carries such positive labels as "intelligent, altruistic, vigorous, outdoing, creative, considerate, energetic, sociable, relaxed, harmonious, and interesting." The fat one is adorned with such adjectives as "compulsive, uncontrolled, base, selfish, greedy, stupid, dull, listless, tense, irritable, dreary, and ugly."

Having such an intensely worthless self-concept is enough to make you want to eat! And eat! And eat!

Along with being in a state of warfare, many people have a tendency to dissect their own bodies into fat and non-fat parts, giving hardly any consideration to the many other qualities of the human body.

How do you feel toward your own body? What words would you use to describe your body? Mostly negative ones, because of your weight?

To develop further self-awareness we present a Body-Image Fantasy that focuses on the range of qualities inherent in human bodies, regardless of whether they are "fat" or "thin."

The Body-Image-Fantasy Exercise

Arrange for some free time. Have someone read this to you, if possible.

We present two sets of instructions for this fantasy. The first is for reading aloud. This is for the person who is reading to you. Following this, we have a paper-and-pencil version for those who are reading the exercise to themselves.

For Reading Aloud

Find a relaxed position. Sit down or lie down, whichever feels more comfortable or convenient for you.

Relax. Stretch three or four times. Breathe deeply for a few minutes. Be aware of the thoughts going through your head. Acknowledge them and then try to let those thoughts leave you. (You can come back to them later.) Be aware of the floor [or couch or chair] beneath you. Are there any tensions in your body? Try to make yourself more comfortable. Take a few more deep breaths.

Now, picture your entire body for a few minutes. Visualize the entire surface from top to bottom.

Keep your attention focused on your body. Now picture the *strongest part* of your body. Where is the strongest part of your body? Get in touch with it. Experience and sense your strongest part. Stay with it a few moments. [The reader should pause one to two minutes now and after each of the following instructions.]

After you have an image of your strongest part, think of the *weakest part* of your body. Let that be central for a while; feel it in all its dimensions, all its qualities, your *weakest part*. [Pause.]

Next, picture the *oldest part* of your body. Take a few minutes to find the *oldest part* of your body. Sense it and experience it for a few moments. [Pause]

Now, think of the *youngest part* of your body. Picture your *youngest part* and get in touch with it. Feel your youngest part for several minutes. [Pause]

Allow plenty of time for each item. It may seem difficult at times to find a particular part, but an answer will come to you.

Then, direct your inner eye toward the *warmest part* of your body. Sense it. Let yourself become fully aware of it. Stay with it a few moments. [Pause] Now, what is the *coldest part* of your body? Get in touch with it. Allow yourself to experience its coldness. [Pause.]

When you're ready, go on to the *smoothest part* of your body. Picture it and sense it. Tune in to how it feels, its special texture. Perhaps touch yourself there, if it's comfortable or possible. [Pause]

After that, become aware of the *roughest part* of your body. Concentrate on your roughest part. Let it be the focal point for a few minutes. [Pause]

Now think of the *hardest part* of your body. Which is your hardest part? Explore it with your mind's eye. Experience its own special quality. [Pause]

Next, what is the most *vulnerable part* of your body, the one most open to hurt and pain? Get in touch with it. Stay with it for a few moments. [Pause]

Then, focus your attention on the *part you most want to change*. Let it be the center of your thoughts and feelings for a few minutes, the part you most want to change. [Pause.]

Now, picture the *part you least want to change*. Which part of your body do you least wish to change? Experience its values and its uniqueness. Give yourself over to the good feeling you get from this. Let it fill your mind. [Pause.]

What is the *most tense part* of your body? Picture it and tune into it. Direct your energy to it. [Pause.]

Now, by contrast, what is the *most relaxed part* of your body? Let it take over for a while, picture it and give it all your attention. Your *most relaxed part*. [Pause.]

Now, focus your attention on the *part you are least proud of*, the one you are *ashamed of*. Find the part you are *least proud of*. Picture it, experience it. [Pause.]

With your mind's eye, picture the *most attractive part* of your body, the part you feel *most proud* of. Explore it in your mind and experience it. [Pause.]

Take several deep breaths. Relax and visualize your entire body once more. Picture all the different parts together, related and connected, and get in touch with the sense of unity of your body. Experience the oneness and wholeness of your body from the surface to the depths. Take several minutes to go over all the parts you focused on during the exercise. [Pause.]

Let your body become reintegrated and consider all the polarities as parts of that unique entity, *your body!* [Pause.]

Allow yourself a few more minutes of experiencing your entire body. Finally, end this exercise by stretching and taking a few deep breaths.

The Written Body-Image-Fantasy Exercise

If you have been reading this exercise to yourself, it is time now to write down all your responses. Do this now, while your recollections are fresh and before reading any further. Too often these ideas will slip away and become unavailable for later study and understanding. Or they will become less real and less intense. This is why we suggest you keep a journal. Writing down events and thoughts relating to your search and exploration of eating, foods, and body awareness gives the information a permanence that can facilitate more self-discoveries later.

Space for answers is provided in the book, but you may prefer to keep your own notes.

There is no time limit; take all the time you wish. For some items, you may have several responses. Write them all down. Then go back over them later to see whether you can narrow down the number to one primary one — or perhaps to two if limiting yourself to one seems too arbitrary.

(Complete each item before going on to the next one)

1. What is the strongest part of your body?

2. What is the weakest part of your body?

3. What is the oldest part of your body?

4. What is the youngest part of your body?

5. What is the warmest part of your body?

6. What is the coldest part of your body?

7. What is the smoothest part of your body?

8. What is the roughest part of your body?

9. What is the hardest part of your body?

10. What is the most vulnerable part of your body?

11. What is the part you most want to change?

12. What is the part you least want to change?

13. What is the most tense part of your body?

14. What is the most relaxed part?

15. What is the part you are least proud of, the part you feel ashamed of?

16. What is the most attractive part of your body, the part you feel most proud of?

Let your body become reintegrated and consider that all the polarities are parts of that unique entity,   *your body!* [Pause.]

Often, people feel surprised after this fantasy. Many are pensive and thoughtful. People frequently find it shakes up their usual negative impression and critical evaluation of their body. This allows a more realistic and accepting view to develop.

Becoming aware of the variety of attributes and qualities of one's own body can mean freedom from the one-dimensional *fat* (ugly)/ *thin* (pretty) concept.

This is especially true for women. In our society a woman's total value as a person is still frequently judged by whether she is "attractive" and has "sex appeal" — and these two attributes are tied to being slender.

A study that received wide newspaper publicity disclosed that obese married women in America have sexual intercourse more frequently than thin women. This might have shaken the idea that being fat and having sex-appeal is incompatible. However, the interpretation of the findings showed the usual cultural bias — fat women were viewed as being more sexually aggressive and initiating sex contact more often *in order to hold onto their mates* . In other words, according to the writer, the fat woman has to act more sexy because she is less sexy! The "thin-me, fat-me" dichotomy carries practical implications.

Many people tend to postpone part of their lives because they consider certain pleasures and activities the sole prerogative of "thinnies." Midway through an intensive week--long vacation-workshop we held in Hawaii, several people wore bathing suits or trunks for the first time in many years. And they swam and played in the water for the first time in a decade, in several instances. They had all been withholding this very real body pleasure from themselves, "until after I get thin."

People similarly restrict their social life "while I'm fat," or don't try for certain jobs (sometimes based on bitter experience), or spend little money on grooming or good-looking clothes "until I get rid of some of this fat." They often order the cheapest meal on the menu because, with all their fat, they "really don't deserve any better."

Postponing living can become a lifestyle, even without a weight problem. One young woman who had postponed much of her life until "after I get thin" came to our workshop *after* she had gotten thin by means of several months of starvation dieting and a marathon fast.

Elaine was twenty-nine, only a fraction over five feet tall, and weighed ninety-eight pounds. She had signed up for the workshop because she was terrified of ever getting fat again.

During discussions and fantasies, Elaine became aware that she hadn't changed the way she related to food — or to herself. She was still critical and unaccepting of her "new" body — except that now her attention was focused on having ugly thighs. For years she perceived nothing but her face when she looked in the mirror. Now she looked at her body, but with a hanging-judge attitude. She located several new areas that her inner jury found guilty of not being thin enough or perfect enough.

Women who accept this thin-vs.-fat value scheme often direct an enormous amount of energy toward achieving the "perfect body" — a goal that can never be reached. Elaine had lived with self-deprecation so long that it had become a familiar and fixed pattern. She was now looking for anything that might be wrong with thin-Elaine. Her liberation from this style can come only by focusing and accepting "me-Elaine."

This chapter has presented you with psychological exercises. We hope they have provided insights into your associations and reactions to food and how you view your body and your eating. The data that comes from this type of self-exploration are usually complex and worthy of additional study. We suggest that you incorporate some of this into your journal so it can aid you in the ongoing process of self-awareness.

12/ *EATING – AWARENESS EXERCISES*

We have found that food-awareness exercises that we have developed over the years are extremely helpful in determining *where* hunger is felt and *what* tastes and textures will really satisfy it.

The purpose behind the exercises which will be presented here and in several following chapters is to develop clarity and focus on a new method for losing weight without diets.

Before providing instructions for the exercises and presenting you with a shopping list — which will be quite unlike any shopping list for overweight people you have ever seen — one word of caution:

Please get the food *now*, before turning the page, before finding out what you will be doing with these mostly forbidden foods. The key to our method, which is successful with most people, is *the experiencing of food in a totally different and new way.*

The exercises are for your own experiments in eating and in relating to food.

Here is the list; please do your shopping *now*:

Food Liberation Shopping List #1

✓ carrot sticks, celery sticks, or radishes (chose two out of these three)
✓ barbecued potato chips
✓ white salted crackers (Waverly or Sunshine Banquet preferred, or Saltines)
✓ a piece of salami
✓ cheese (any fairly mild soft cheese. Suggestions: Monterey Jack, Muenster, Fontina)
✓ 2 whole dill pickles
✓ an empty medium-sized paper bag.

Try to wait until after you have obtained all the above items before you go on to the next section.

•

Assemble these items and arrange for some free, undisturbed time. If you have a friend or spouse who is *genuinely* supportive of your aims and with whom you feel *fully* comfortable, have that person read the instructions to you as you do the exercises, one by one.

Please note that we said "genuinely." If the other person is likely to be critical ("Do you really think eating this junk will help you lose weight?") or if you would feel self-conscious or embarrassed in his or her presence, forget it. You are far better off reading through the entire exercise once yourself, and then rereading it, paragraph by paragraph, as you follow instructions.

You can also consider having two or three close friends, all with eating or weight problems, join you to go through the food exercises together. Whichever style is comfortable and most convenient for you is the method to use.

We want to make it clear before we start that this exercise is in no way intended to turn you on to certain foods (like rabbit food) or turn you *off* others (like potato chips or salami). It is simply an exploration of sensations that can help you toward a more efficient way of obtaining pleasure and satisfaction in eating, and these are basic to our long-range permanent-weight-loss program.

One of the behaviors shared by many overeaters is a style of eating. There is a rapid, robotlike quality to it; food is processed rather than experienced. People who eat in this manner develop emotional and sensory calluses — very often on their fingers, or lips, or tongue, or maybe one whole side of the mouth — and these parts fail to transmit to the brain any signal that denotes a real experience of the food being ingested.

The first exercise is designed to help you become aware of this process.

The Rabbit-Food Exercise

To start the exercise, break off a piece of carrot or celery or pick up a radish.

Which hand are you now holding it in? Feel it by rolling it between your fingers and letting it slip to the palm of your hand.

Transfer it to the opposite hand. *Don't look at it; just feel it.* Close your eyes for a few moments. Feel the texture, the temperature. Does it seem different in this hand from the hand you first held it in? Does it seem bigger or smaller, rougher or smoother, colder or warmer, familiar or strange? More sensitive or less? These are all qualities some group members have reported as being different in one hand than in the other.

Now switch it back to the original hand, which is undoubtedly your "preferred" hand. Most people have one hand that is definitely their preferred one, and the very simple act of changing hands can create new awareness of the qualities of many foods.

Next, bring the food up to your mouth *as if* to take a bite. Don't bite it yet, just hold it there.

Where are you? What is your angle of attack? Center of the mouth, left side, right side, food pointed straight in or coming up at an angle?

Just as they have a preferred hand, most people have a preferred angle of attack; and just as the preferred hand may have become callused and devoid of sensation, so may the lips and the part of the mouth that generally receive the food. This may seem like a very minute detail, but if you want to change a lifelong eating pattern, it is essential to break the whole eating process down into just such minute components.

✶ Next, take the piece of food in the *unaccustomed* hand and bring it to your mouth at an unaccustomed angle and bite off a piece. Let it rest in your mouth a moment. What does it feel like? Explore it. Move it around a bit, run your tongue over it. What is it like?

192

Now bite it in half. Do you feel a spurt of flavor? Is there a different inner texture? Explore the inner surface, and compare it to the outer texture.

You have seen science-fiction movies where a giant chews up something. The whole screen is filled with a deliberately moving pair of jaws. Imagine yourself to be that giant and chew in just such a slow-motion, deliberate, and even exaggerated way. Study the motion of your teeth, your jaws. Where is your tongue?

When the food is really ground up, move it to the front of the mouth and hold it there a moment, then press it against the roof of your mouth, extracting all flavor possible.

Now, either swallow it or spit in into the paper bag. That's right: Try spitting it out.

Ever since our days in the high chair, we have been so conditioned to eat politely that we have lost track of some of our options. Of course you wouldn't spit out food on the middle of a banquet table, but in your own home and in privacy, why not spit out something that is disagreeable? You not only have the right to *choose* the food you want, you also have the right to *reject* that which you don't want. You can exercise both rights. We're not suggesting that you spit out food as a habit — and certainly *not* as a way of losing weight. But we especially would like you to experience it in terms of "How does it feel to waste food — to throw it away, to reject it?"

Now pick another piece of rabbit food, a different kind from the one you used the first time around. Break off a piece and repeat the whole exercise — that is, let the *unaccustomed* hand bring it to the *unaccustomed* side of the mouth, bite off a piece, and proceed as above, starting with the starred paragraph.

After completing this part of the exercise, take a small break. Walk around if you feel like it. You don't have to do all the exercises in one sitting; you can come back to them when the book hums to you. When you have the privacy, time, and inclination.

The Potato-Chip Exercise

Ready to go on? Open the bag of potato chips and take out one unbroken chip. What hand is it in? Probably the same one you used for picking up the rabbit food.

Switch the chip to the unaccustomed hand (or have you already put it there?). Smell the chip. This, again, is something rarely done, because it isn't polite. It's a peculiar quirk of our culture that it is fine to walk into a house and tell the hostess, "Something smells delicious." Yet it is considered boorish to pick up a fork-full at the table and sniff it.

Think of how often we tell children, "There's nothing wrong with your food — stop smelling it, just eat it." The association is that smelling implies criticism. Yet, great chefs always smell and taste their food.

The olfactory qualities of food are immensely important to full appreciation and enjoyment. Physiological studies have shown that taste is really partly smell. We have all had the experience of finding during a bad cold that nothing tastes right. Unable to smell the food, we are partially unable to taste it, and our awareness of it and our pleasure are diminished.

Studies have shown that, deprived of vision and smell, people cannot differentiate between many foods — between applesauce and mashed potatoes, between wine and lemonade. Try it sometime. *Close your eyes and hold your nose. Then have someone feed you a variety of foods. You will be surprised at how few you will identify correctly.*

Wine connoisseurs know the importance of smell and freely practice the art of sniffing. If you cannot bring yourself to sniff food in public, at least allow yourself this pleasure and exploration in private eating.

Now: Forget your good manners even further and lick the potato chip. Consider that sensation, then smell once more. Any change? Often a food that is slightly moistened releases stronger fragrances.

Now another lick. Some foods are primarily carriers of flavor: They serve as vehicles for a spice or seasoning. It is worthwhile to check this out. If, for instance, you are one of the people to whom the barbecue *taste* of the chip is the most important and satisfying part, why eat potato chips at all? There are much more efficient ways of satisfying this taste preference. You might even enjoy pure barbecue flavoring. How aware are you of your *specific* preferences — and how *efficient* are you in getting your preferences?

Your licked chip is probably something less than appetizing-looking by now. Throw it into the paper bag.

Take out a new potato chip, let the unaccustomed hand take it to the mouth at an unaccustomed angle, and this time take a big bite, *but don't chew.* You may feel impatient and feel like you are teasing your own taste buds. Remember, later you can eat the whole bag, but right now you are exploring.

Keep the bite of potato chip in the front of your mouth and just let it dissolve there; then press it against the roof of your mouth to get the juices out. Turn the soft potato pulp over and over until there is no flavor left. What does it feel like? Is it pleasant or unpleasant? Many people find it unpalatable; others enjoy it.

Now, either swallow it or spit it out. Was it easier to spit it out? Observe your own reactions to this process of spitting it out, if you did that.

On to another chip. This time, you are the slow-motion giant again. Visualize grinding up that chip slowly and methodically; now, painstakingly demolish it, but don't swallow yet. What is the taste like? How does it compare to the sensations you got from the dissolved chip? How does it compare to only licking the chip? Check it out, then either swallow it or spit it out.

Take another chip, only this time chew it up as fast as you can; really race through it. Is this the way you usually eat potato chips? How does it compare with the other two experiments? Do you get more enjoyment from the texture or flavor this way or in one of the other ways?

How about the taste? Once again, you can swallow it or spit it out.

Consider the whole potato chip experience now. What was it you really liked? Take a few minutes now to review it.

Whatever it is, do you think potato chips are the most efficient way of getting this particular food satisfaction?

Remember, this is no attempt to turn you off potato chips — or anything else. If you really like the combination of crunchiness, saltiness, barbecue flavor, and potato pulp, barbecued potato chips will give you a very satisfying eating experience.

But if it's the chewing that you really want, there are more efficient, pleasurable foods for that. Check out more efficient ways of satisfying that need for a moment. Nuts or beef jerky come to our mind.

If it's the saltiness, how about licking a bit of salt? We know that animals do it, and kids do it until they are taught it's impolite.

We have already talked of the barbecue flavor. But if the potatoiness is what you most enjoy, consider whether you would not get greater pleasure and true eating satisfaction out of eating the real thing, that is, real potatoes. Ponder the possibilities: baked potato, hash browns, French fries, pan-fried potatoes, mashed potatoes, dumplings, potato pancakes.

If you really love the potato quality of the chip, check out which of the dishes we just mentioned gets at the essence of that thing called "potato" for you.

That dish would be the best choice for you — the most efficient way to satisfy a specific hunger.

Take another break or, if you wish, finish the exercise tomorrow. Remember, there is no success-or-failure element in these experiments. They are simply an aid to your checking yourself out. You might even feel like taking down a few notes about your feelings and thoughts right now. You might want to repeat the exercise in a few weeks, and it might be interesting to read your own reactions. You would probably find quite a few differences. As we mentioned earlier, we suggest a journal for those who are so inclined — a journal of your reactions and feelings as you become more aware of tastes and preferences.

At any rate, the crackers are next.

The Cracker Exercise

Pick one up and change it from hand to hand. Feel it and smell it. Lick it and smell again. Do you pick up the butter flavor and smell? Salt? What else? Is it appealing? Which aspect appeals?

Proceed much as you did with the potato chips, first taking a small bite from the *unaccustomed* hand (notice how often you skip over to using the "automatic" hand) and at an unaccustomed angle, keeping it in the front of the mouth and letting it dissolve. Don't chew it. Press it against the roof of the mouth and extract juices, then explore the pulp. Finally, either swallow it or spit it out.

Next do the slow-motion-giant routine. Give yourself plenty of time to explore all tastes, textures, and sensations at every step. Take a small slow motion chew, then move the pulp to the center part of your mouth and, pressing with your tongue against the roof of your mouth, extract the flavor before going on to the next bite. Now chew one bite fast and contrast the sensations. What's your preference?

Finally, take one cracker and eat it in little tiny nibbles, like a mouse, doing all the chewing with your front teeth only, turning it so you just nibble off the edge. Does this feel good, or do you prefer the back chewing? Again, we have been taught that it isn't good manners to chew in front. Yet, to a good number of people much needed oral-dental satisfaction comes from front chewing. These people often chew and eat very large quantities of food just to get some front chewing experience — a very inefficient way to obtain satisfaction.

Others, of course, like the feeling of a full mouth. For them, chewing foods, such as crackers, are really wasted. In the bread category, a slice or two of fairly soft-textured bread would probably be far more efficient. These people might also consider whether they aren't cheating themselves when they eat toast. Plain bread might be far more enjoyable. If you are one of these people, get plain breads and don't be intimidated by menus or waiters who might inform you that such and such "comes toasted." It's your order and your money. Tell them you want plain bread.

The people who enjoy chewing should do just the opposite, that is, insist on getting the crackers or toast or hard rolls or ends of the loaf they really enjoy. Many people have told us that they overeat on pizza, because even after they feel full the flavor and the chewing are irresistible. There is one solution: Chew it and spit it out. This has nothing to do with the old wisecrack, too often heard by the obese, "You can eat anything you want, so long as you don't swallow it." It is simply an assertion of your right to the satisfaction you want without having to pay for it by enduring the unpleasantness of an over-full stomach.

Review what happened so far. Try jotting down a few notes right now.

The Cheese Exercise

Next, we move on to cheese. First smell it, then lick it. Change hands and run it over your lips. Do you like the soft, smooth feeling? Does it make you want to feel that same smoothness in your mouth?

Suck on the cheese. Again, this may sound odd and rude, but it may turn out to be a pleasurable sensation, even though you may have been scolded for doing just that as a child. ("Don't lick or suck your food!")

In general, cheese is not an efficient chewing food. If you are looking for a chewing experience, cheese obviously couldn't give you the full satisfaction you would derive from other foods, such as nuts, pretzels, or hard toast.

But if you are a true cheese lover, or cheese "freak," the smell and textural sensation derived from sucking probably are highly enjoyable to you.

Incidentally, if you love butter, cheese eaten in our different manner may also prove highly satisfying. Quite a few people in our workshops reported that they found a mild, soft cheese even more pleasurable and filling than butter. Butter, by its very nature, melts and disappears so fast that it gives only a very brief sensation, and, once swallowed, is gone.

A creamy cheese will melt in the mouth, too, only much more slowly, so the taste and the pleasure last longer. Moreover, even with a mild cheese, there is some residual taste around the teeth or palate that lingers long after the cheese is gone. Check it out sometime, if you are a butter lover.

As you will see as we progress, we believe that the sensual enjoyment food provides is a valid experience, and that it is psychologically very important.

The issue becomes: How can you find the most precise way of pleasuring yourself with food?

Take a medium-size bite of cheese and let it rest in the front of your mouth until it seems to start to melt. Don't bite; just press it against the roof of the mouth with your tongue. This is similar to what we did with the crackers. Let the cheese warm to your mouth's temperature; let it melt and suck the flavor down your mouth and into your throat. Now, take another bite and move the cheese into one cheek, so it rests a moment outside your teeth.

Try the same on the other side. Let your tongue work it around in the cheek area till it's gone. Then let the tongue explore the areas where it was. Pick up the aftertaste.

Take another bite, but this time keep it all in the lower part of your mouth. Lean on it with your tongue; work it around until it is gone. One more bite, and this time try once again to let it melt in the very center of your mouth.

Which of the three ways appeals most to you? You'll notice that with both cheese and crackers we've suggested experimenting with ways of eating; you suck, "gum," extract flavor, allowing the food to melt in your mouth. For chewing and biting — which are different sensations for different moods and needs — obviously cheese and crackers offer little resistance, and may not be an efficient food.

Take another break, or, once again, if you think this is enough for now, postpone the rest of the exercises till tomorrow.

The Salami Exercise

Salami is one of the many sandwich foods that some people are never fully aware of. That is to say, they may like salami-and-cheese sandwiches, or salami sandwiches with mustard and pickle, but the tastes are always such a mixture that they have no very clear mental taste picture of salami.

It is entirely possible that it is that very mélange of tastes that appeals to you. There are true Poor Boy, Hero, or Dagwood sandwich fans. But a great many of these taste combinations are simply routine habitual patterns. From the time Mother put sandwiches into your lunch box as a first-grader, you have probably been confronted with many of these combinations as though there were a law that this is the way certain foods are eaten. It's certainly worth checking out what you really like.

We once had a German engineer at our Institute who said his great weakness were *braunschweiger* sandwiches. A delicatessen near his office had very good *braunschweiger* and made sandwiches on rye bread with caraway seeds, combining the *braunschweiger* with several thin slices of cheese, pickles, lettuce, and a generous scoop of mayonnaise.

The engineer picked up eight to ten of these a day. He would eat three or four for lunch and the rest throughout the evening as a bedtime snack. In our eating exercises, he was able to establish that he did indeed love the *braunschweiger* but that it was much more satisfying to him without bread, without cheese, and especially without mayonnaise, which, in pure form, he found he genuinely disliked.

Part of the change in his eating pattern was that he started to buy *braunschweiger* by the half-pound, as well as jars of the delicatessen shop's spicy pickles. He ate the sausage with pickles for lunch. He allowed himself to eat all he wanted, which was generally about half of the half-pound package. He frequently had more *braunschweiger* and pickles in the evening but, more often than not, it was instead of dinner rather than as an after-dinner snack. This was not a diet attempt. Rather, he had found that very often he was eating a big dinner without feeling satisfied. The dinner tasted good, but it wasn't really the food that was humming to him.

Also, from the back of his memory something came back to him that he had totally forgotten: His mother sometimes had served thin slices of *braunschweiger* and fresh radishes to his father and his friends when they got together for a beer on Saturday morning.

He tried this combination and loved it, so radishes — which he had despised as diety rabbit food — became part of his most enjoyable eating experience.

Pick up a chunk of salami and smell it. How does it smell to you? Have you ever really slowly smelled salami before? You might get another kind of salami or bologna and compare the smells. Now change hands and lick it. Try to verbalize the taste and the tactile sensations you pick up: smooth, slightly wet, uneven surface, salty, smoky, a bacony taste — whatever message you get.

Change hands again and slide the salami slowly across your lips. What sensation do you pick up now? Lick your lips. Most of us miss out on the unique experience of licking a food like salami.

Next, take a good-size bite, but *don't chew it.* Let it warm up in the center of your mouth; then roll it around, making it rotate. Is that pleasurable?

Now, "gum" it. Pretend you are toothless and try to extract flavor by working on it with gums and tongue. Investigate it with your tongue some more.

We have found that many people never stop to explore their own tongue capabilities in either food or sex, and never discover what a marvelously intricate part of the body the tongue is. There are approximately three thousand taste buds located in tiny, wart-like papillae on the human tongue, but they are by no means all alike. The buds at the very back of the tongue are sensitive to bitter tastes, the ones at the tip to sweet, and the ones on the side to sour. The very center of the tongue has no buds, so no taste sensation is experienced there, but pressure is felt there.

We hope that while reading this you have thoroughly explored the piece of salami with your tongue.

Next, lean your teeth gently against it and pierce it slightly. Is there a burst of flavor? If so, exactly what is it like? Spicy, smoky? Can you feel it in your throat as it trickles down? On which side of the mouth is it now? Change it over to the opposite side and start grinding it up, very slowly, very deliberately. Then, either swallow it or spit it out.

Next, take another chunk and chew it in tiny bites as fast as you can, as much as possible with your *front teeth only.* How does that feel, by comparison? How do you feel about salami at this point?

Some people have a feeling of satisfaction, the joy of a new pleasant discovery. They savor the aftertaste, remembering the taste and flavor experience they just had — the saltiness, the smoky quality, the smooth, oily aspect of salami, the experience of feeling the separate tiny morsels of meat and fat, of now and then picking up the essential taste of a spice.

Others experience much the same, but they find they do not savor it. To them, the texture may now seem unpleasantly coarse, the flavor of smoke and spices biting, the saltiness an irritant, the oiliness slightly nauseating.

Get in touch with your own reactions. Where are you now in relation to salami?

The Pickle Exercise

After a brief pause and maybe a sip of water, move onto one of the pickles. Pickles are considered trimmings, extraneous items, hardly food at all, yet they are a unique food with flavor and texture of strong identity. To us, they are an overlooked source of legitimate eating pleasure.

If you really like pickles, there is no reason why you should relegate them to the trimming-only category and why you should contaminate their taste and texture with all sorts of other stuff. Eat pickles all by themselves. We have found many latent pickle freaks who really can enjoy pickles plain or in pickle sandwiches.

For our next exercise, cut a thin slice from the end of one of the pickles. Smell it, then change hands. Run it across your lips. How does it feel? Cool, slippery, rubbery? Take a lick — what taste components do you pick up? Briny, sour, dill taste, spicy? Which of these do you find appealing? Or unattractive?

Put the slice in your mouth and let it rest inside the front teeth against the lower lip. Move it around a bit. Does it feel squeaky?

Press it against the roof of the mouth with your tongue, then let it slide into your jaw way in back past your wisdom teeth and apply jaw pressure.

Next, pierce it gently with your teeth, for a burst of flavor. What kind of flavor? Pierce it again slightly with your front teeth.

Now try the other side and let it rest between the molars, in the back.

Finally, play "big giant" and chew the remains in extreme slow motion.

Slowly feel the texture as you chew. What other sensation remains?

Swallow the pickle slice or spit it out, then check out how your mouth feels now. With your tongue, explore your lips, and the roof of your mouth. Is the aftertaste pleasant?

Many overeaters, especially when eating a "non-dietary" food, hurry through the eating process so fast that they never experience such sensations as an initial taste, then a flavor burst, then an aftertaste. There is no lingering, loving experience for them. The guilt feelings which we discussed earlier get in the way. If this has been your approach — if you always eat as if this were the last time you will ever have this forbidden food and you had better demolish it fast *(before* somebody sees, *before* you have second thoughts, *before* someone might take it away) — check out how you like the sensations you are experiencing in this exercise.

Next, pick up the rest of the pickle. Smell it. Feel it. Lick it. Put it in the *unaccustomed* hand (or have you done so already?) and chose a different angle of attack, then take a big bite. Chew it as quickly as you can, process it, and swallow it or spit it out.

Which way of eating gives you more of an awareness of the essence of a pickle? Which is more pleasurable?

Either way of eating is legitimate and valid, and we are not trying to make slow eaters out of everybody. But you should be aware of the options and then choose the way that brings you maximum enjoyment and satisfaction.

Check out how you feel right now. How much time has gone by since you started the exercise, or this particular part? Are you hungry? Would you like more of any of the foods we have exercised with? Would you like something completely different?

The Sandwich Exercise

Before we conclude, we would like to try one more step. Make an open face sandwich of a cracker, a slice of pickle, a slice of salami, and a slice of cheese. Take a small bite and hold it in your mouth a moment without chewing. How does this feel? Start chewing very deliberately. Does any one component of the sandwich stand out? Pleasantly or as too dominant? Chew with your eyes closed. What is your reaction?

Now extract the salami and cheese and take another small bite of the pickle-cracker combination. How do you like the pickle sandwich?

Go through the same process with all the components, taking new crackers or slices of food as needed.

How do you like a salami-and-cracker sandwich? Or cheese-and-cracker, or salami-and-cheese, or cheese-and-pickle, or salami-and-cheese-and-cracker, or pickle and cheese and salami? In other words, experiment. Would you just as well have them all together again or would you prefer each component by itself? Which double combination, if any, really turns you on? Is there one or the other component that you really don't care for at all? There's no need to be bound by any food conventions — you can select only those taste sensations you prefer.

This concludes this particular exercise. We will outline others later in the book, but you may also wish to duplicate it on your own with different foods, particularly some favorite food that you may want to get to know and enjoy better. Your preferred binging food would be an excellent choice. As you can see, we are suggesting a long delicious affair with food, rather than the rape that frequently occurs.

Before we move on, we would like you once more to consider the combinations of food you have just tried. If you have found that there were aspects to this combination of cheese, cracker, salami, and pickle that you didn't like, consider some other combinations that you commonly eat. Focus your awareness on these combinations. What turns you on in a toasted bacon, lettuce, tomato, and mayonnaise sandwich? The mayonnaise and bacon? Or the toast and tomato? Find out and eat *it*.

At the Institute, we keep running into the problem of people eating certain combinations, not because they really enjoy them, but simply because certain foods are customarily presented in a certain grouping: bacon and eggs, pie with ice cream, toast with butter, pork with applesauce, spaghetti with meat sauce, steak and potatoes, soup and crackers.

All of these combinations are intrinsically acceptable and palatable — *if* they are what you really want. But many people need to stop and reexamine these habitually eaten food combinations and determine their own precise preferences. Allow yourself to eat exactly the combinations you like; insist on them.

If you like a doughnut with your scrambled eggs, that's the emotionally satisfying thing to eat. Whose business is it except yours? If you like an onion sandwich on raisin bread, fine. Potato salad for breakfast, pie for lunch, hot oatmeal and orange juice for supper? Why not?

We had another sandwich freak at the institute; unlike the German engineer, he ate sandwiches chiefly for the mayonnaise in them.

He ate great quantities of hamburgers, cold meat sandwiches, tuna salad, and the like — which he discovered he really didn't crave. After he explored his cravings, he installed a refrigerator in his car (he was a successful importer and could well afford this little luxury). Now, instead of racing away from the office at 5:00 P.M., panting for sandwiches, visualizing himself at home, he sits in the garage for a moment, gets out his box of crackers and his jar of mayonnaise, and has a couple of mayonnaise-cracker sandwiches. The sandwich shop that's located halfway between his office and his home has lost a customer, but he is a far more content (and, incidentally, thinner) man.

As we've suggested earlier, one key to permanent weight loss is a feeling of liberation regarding food — a casting off of the bonds that restricted you to certain times to eat, certain limited types of food, certain combinations, etc.

A sense of freedom toward food is critical for lasting changes in eating behavior, and these exercises are part of the process.

13/ *DRINKING– AWARENESS EXERCISES*

Please follow the same pattern you used with the eating exercises, arranging for free time and a companion you feel at ease with (if that is possible), and do your shopping before you proceed. Teetotalers can skip the alcoholic part. Also, omit any beverages that you never drink or never feel like drinking — for example, if you never drink either tea or coffee, omit that category. If you dislike beer, skip it. However, if you do drink alcoholic beverages, but have never really tried liqueurs, for example, we suggest you buy at least one or two of the small sample-size bottles which most liquor stores carry and use them in the experiments that follow.

The Liberated Drinker's Shopping List

✓ 8 ounces chilled fruit juice (your choice)
✓ 1 can or bottle of plain sparkling water
✓ 1 can beer
✓ 1 glass wine (your choice)
✓ 1 glass liqueur (your choice)
✓ Ingredients for making your favorite mixed drink
✓ Straws
✓ Ice cubes

The Fruit Juice Exercise

In our workshops we use apple juice. Orange juice, pineapple juice, or whatever your favorite fruit juice is will do equally well.

Pour a small amount of juice into a glass. Smell the juice. Then take a small sip and drink as you ordinarily do.

Next, take a straw. Barely hold the straw between your lips and take a tiny sip, trying to let it trickle into the front of your mouth, and keep it there. How does drinking through a straw contrast with sipping in your usual manner? What flavors are you aware of? What is dominant, the sweetness or the tangy or tart quality? Take several more sips with the straw, trying to keep the beverage in the front of your mouth for a few moments.

Next, try to use your tongue as a valve that regulates flow. That means you take sips through the straw; shut off the flow every so often with the tip of your tongue pressed against the top of the straw; then release it again.

Is it fun to do that? How is the taste experience?

Now put the straw on one side of your mouth and take a sip. (The straw is held between your teeth on one side and you draw the juice up.) It's a bit awkward, but focus on how this feels and tastes.

Which side did you drink on? Once again, this is probably your preferred side. It may have some of the taste calluses we discussed earlier. Therefore, try the same exercise on the other side. Can you pick up any differences? Is there more sensation and enjoyment, or less? Comments usually include "no difference" or "colder," "tastier," "less sweet," "more appleish," "sweeter," and "more satisfying."

People are often quite unaware of being left-or right-cheek drinkers. It's possible to increase pleasurable sensations by consciously shifting sides when you drink.

Now, take a sip and swish the fruit juice through your mouth. Swish another sip back and forth along the sides of your mouth. This makes some fluids extremely flavorful.

For the next few sips, play with the straw. Wrap your tongue around it; hold it so you sip mostly through your front teeth; alternate long sips and very short ones. Explore the various sensations; try to determine which, if any, is the most pleasurable.

The next exercise is somewhat complicated and can be uncomfortable if not done carefully. Put the straw as far back toward your throat as you can without choking, up against your palate. Suck the straw and the juice will squirt far back into the top of your throat. Don't choke, but at the same time try to get the juice directly to your throat, bypassing the front of your mouth.

What are your reactions? Some people say they miss the flavor this way; others are startled at how good this feels. This is an area that often gets cheated, especially with cold drinks, because in the conventional way of drinking the liquid is no longer ice-cold by the time it reaches your throat, having been warmed by your mouth. Yet many people crave the cold sensation in their throat. (Many milkshake freaks savor and relish the cold-sweet experience in this area.)

We have often found people who overeat sweet-cold foods because they are trying to obtain this particular sensa-

213

tion at the back of their throat. But for this need, food is inefficient. Use of a straw can deliver the *undiluted* sensation with accuracy. This is, incidentally, not an unusual style of drinking. Spaniards using the leather *bota* literally squirt wine right into their throats, and good old-fashioned American corn whiskey is traditionally drunk this way, jug on the shoulder, head tilted way back.

Next, we would like you to try something you were probably scolded for doing as a child — gargling with your drink.

Try out the two basic styles of gargling: (1) aerating the drink vigorously and making a sound in the typical way; (2) without phonating, gargling almost silently.

This is a further way of getting in touch with the throat and its sensitivities. We usually focus on this area only in distress, when there is something wrong, when we have a sore throat. Experience your healthy, well throat. How does the gargling feel? Are you more aware of the sweetness or tartness of the juice? Does the gargling release a burst of aroma? Can you smell as well as taste the juice?

Do another "kid thing": Blow through the straw and make bubbles in the glass. How about the fragrance now? Any difference in taste?

Then, squeeze the straw a little flat between your teeth so only a small amount of liquid can get through and you have to suck hard to get even that. Fix the straw so you have to use "muscle" to get the juice. Do this for a few minutes. How does it feel to use these sucking muscles? These are muscles that are denied full use in most everyday eating or drinking, yet they are another source of sensory input and of pleasure.

One workshop participant became worried about herself at this point and asked, "Does enjoying sucking like this prove my orality?" Do such labels as "oral-dependent," "infantile," and "oral personality" come to your mind? As we discussed earlier, such generalized labels are meaningless. They are used as put-downs and as pseudopsychological diagnoses. Enjoying sucking sensations mean nothing more than that this is a pleasant sensation for you — and millions of others. It is a sensation you are entitled to experience.

Add an ice cube to the juice that remains in the glass and wait a few moments until it has cooled the juice. Pour some warmer juice into a separate glass. We'd like to have you contrast the two.

Take a sip of the colder juice and then a sip from the other glass. How do the two compare? Do you like your juice ice cold or do you get more flavor from the warmer juice? To some people the warmer juice is sweeter, sharper, more fruity, and more filling. To others the warmer juice tastes dull, flat, even "like rotten fruit." Where are you?

Many people give little thought to their options. They drink their coffee and tea hot, their fruit juices and soft drinks chilled, their beer and champagne ice cold, their red wine at room temperature, their white and rosé wine cool, their brandy from glasses that are slightly warmed, and their highballs and some other mixed drinks with ice — and all this mostly because "that's the way you drink it."

Who says that's the way *you* have to drink it? Probably the majority do get the greatest flavor experience and pleasure from all these beverages at those temperatures. But not everybody.

In checking it out, you may find that you are unable to taste (or fully experience) any flavor if a beverage is at either extreme — very hot or very cold. To others, anything lukewarm is unpalatable. And "lukewarm" often includes room temperature. If any of these people follow conventional methods and drink beverages at temperatures that don't hum to them, they are bound to lose out on much, if not all, pleasure from the beverage.

Over drinking can result from any unsatisfactory state, whether wrong temperature, taste, or even container. One of our participants told us how she is used to drinking coffee out of a large ceramic coffee mug. During a vacation trip she was amazed to discover that her sudden overeating at breakfast was due to a real dissatisfaction with the size of hotel coffee cups. She was feeling frustrated and cheated of good coffee sensations and taking it out by extra eating. The obvious solution was to buy a coffee mug of the type she was used to, and carry it with her.

It's fairly easy to get coffee, tea and fruit juices the way you want them. You can let the hot beverages sit until they cool down, and the cold ones until they warm up. Even putting an ice cube into a cup of steaming hot coffee is considered only mildly odd.

But when it comes to alcoholic beverages, there is a real problem. Would you be embarrassed to order red dinner wine chilled? Have you ever tried warm beer? Or drinking beer (cold or warm) through a straw? Have you had chilled cognac?

One of our favorites is putting an ice cube in wine or champagne.

Englishmen and many New Zealanders generally drink their beer unchilled, particularly stout. And many Frenchmen mix their red *vin ordinaire* with cold water at lunch and dinnertime.

Have you ever tried drinking half red wine and half carbonated water? College students call it "dormitory champagne." Also, one of our favorites is three parts apple juice mixed with one part carbonated water. This creates a bubbly apple taste that is delicious.

Carbonated water can be a unique and pleasant sensation in the mouth and throat. If you drink Coke, 7-Up, or other carbonated drinks, experiment with carbonated water to intensify the taste of other liquids, such as juices.

The Beer Exercise

Try drinking beer using the same exercises as the ones for the fruit juice. Include a cold/warm test if it sounds at all interesting to you. Also, experiment with pouring some beer into a glass, allowing lots of foam to form. Many beer drinkers try to avoid a big head. But try using a straw to drink the foamy part. Then try the clear part. Do you like it? Notice any taste difference?

It may seem odd to drink beer through a straw. But straws intensify flavor for most people, and pinpoint the delivery to a narrow band of taste registers.

With the beer, be especially attentive to the aftertaste.

We have one more suggestion concerning beer. If you usually eat pretzels or chips with beer, try licking some plain salt as you drink. Use a style similar to that used by Mexicans to drink tequila: You lick the outside of your clenched fist, between thumb and index finger, sprinkle salt on it, and then lick the salt off as you drink. Does beer have a different after-taste if you omit salty foods or plain salt? What does the salt do to the flavor of beer for you?

COFFEE OR TEA "CHAIN DRINKING"

If you are a coffee or tea "chain drinker," you might experiment and explore other coffees and teas. Exotic coffees are easily available, so you can try coffee with chicory, Kona coffee, French roast, and Mocha Java, to name a few. Have you tried Viennese-style coffee with whipped cream? It can be the ultimate coffee experience for some. If you like cream and sugar in your coffee, consider trying a scoop of ice cream instead. Or try heating the milk or cream before adding it to the coffee. (This is traditionally done throughout Mexico.) It does taste different!

Tea drinkers might try the wide range of popular English blends, such as English Breakfast and Earl Grey, or some of the more exotic Oriental ones like green tea and Mu tea. Many of these are available in tea bags for convenience. Mint and other herb teas also offer a great variety of aromas that you might enjoy exploring, as do such special blends as Constant Comment, an orange-flavored tea.

The Liqueur-Awareness Exercise

It's time to try several awareness exercises with your liqueur. Take a small sip and bring the liqueur to the front of your mouth, between the front of your teeth and the inside of your lips. Try especially to keep it in the upper half of your mouth. This can be an area of sharp sensory awareness. Is it pleasant for you? Or too much? Too sweet? Too strong? Try drinking liqueurs on the rocks. Does the coldness interfere with aroma and taste? Or does it provide a blend of sensations you enjoy?

Experiment with a drink of liqueur on some occasions when "something sweet" hums to you. Liqueurs can be more efficient than candy or desserts, especially if you are too tense to experience food fully. The liqueur is a highly concentrated drink that not only relaxes but whose intense, sweet flavors satisfy.

The Cocktail Exercise

Do you have a favorite mixed drink? If so, we would like you to do a drinking awareness exercise with it. Assemble all the ingredients *without* mixing them yet. (For the purposes of this exercise, already premixed bottled cocktails, or the dry mix packets to which you add only the appropriate liquor, will not work.)

We will outline the exercise for the martini drinker. If this isn't your thing, substitute whatever the ingredients of your favorite drink are. The principles are the same.

First, an exercise especially for the olive. Mix a small drink and place an olive in it. Let the olive soak. Try enjoying the olive in a different way. Suck the pitted center of the olive and chew the pimento in small bites. Then put the olive back in your drink and from time to time suck the olive's flavor. This may not be considered polite, but it can be fun; it's a little like dunking doughnuts in coffee.

Now, pour small amounts of gin and vermouth into two separate, fresh glasses.

Take a sip of vermouth and hold it in the front of your mouth. Check out the vermouth much as you checked out fruit juice: Swish it around in your mouth. Try other exercises — gargling, using a straw, etc. Do the same with the gin. How do these drinks taste separately? Some people feel it's sacrilegious, others find it interesting.

We find that reactions vary greatly. How did gin feel on the tip of your tongue? Did you like it in your cheek, or did it give you a sharp and vivid sensation there, or a sting? How did it feel in your throat?

Now repeat the above using ice — two separate glasses, with vermouth on the rocks and gin on the rocks.

Once in a while, someone who considered himself a staunch martini drinker finds out that he really doesn't like gin very much. If that is the case, experiment. At the next opportunity, sample a vodka martini, or maybe vermouth over ice with a twist of lemon. Only experimentation will help you find the most satisfying drink for your palate, and that's a basic human right: finding the precise drinks and foods for maximum pleasuring.

Other people discover unexpectedly that they like gin a lot and that they like it best alone, without the vermouth. They can reap a bonus besides increased pleasure from their drink: In most bars, a shot of gin is considerably cheaper than a mixed drink.

Audrey, a twenty-seven-year-old Sacramento telephone supervisor, found that she enjoyed gin by itself and without ice. "But I don't know if I'd have the nerve to order it that way in a bar. That sounds like a wino — drinking straight booze." She finally did drink a martini minus vermouth at her own place when only her boyfriend was there. She decided to go with it this way always.

If you found your fondness for martinis confirmed, you might add a few experiments of your own at another time, such as: varying the proportions of gin and vermouth; despite the *Bartender's Guide* recommendations, chilling all ingredients and the glass as well, but skipping the ice; having it on the rocks; using dry sherry in place of vermouth.

One man found that a sake martini — gin with just a few drops of the traditional Japanese rice wine — became his favorite.

Also, you might try different brands of gin and vermouth. There is a wide range of flavor variations between the liquors marketed as gin, and also in vermouth from Italy, France, the U.S., etc. Fortunately, the most expensive is not necessarily the one most enjoyable for you. But if a Tanqueray martini hums to you, there is a good chance that a martini made with the house gin of your local discount liquor store will leave you dissatisfied. Your budget may not give you the option of using an expensive brand all the time. But if at all possible, don't settle for what's second-best on your own scale of taste values.

We have explored not only tastes, but many different modes of drinking. To gain maximum satisfaction from drinking, it is essential to stick with the modes that are most enjoyable to you as an individual drinker — even if they are "far out." We recall the experience of one friend of ours, a slender ex-smoker, who loves to gargle with martinis before dinner to get the sensation into her upper throat.

"How do you do that in a restaurant?" we inquired.

"Simple — you pretend you are admiring the chandeliers."

Skol! Prosit! Cheers! *L`Charon! A votre sante!* Bottoms up! Try it — you may like it!

14/ THE SENSUOUS MOUTH – AN AWARENESS EXERCISE

The psychological calluses are so strong in many people that they have little awareness of their mouths except as a tunnel between the outside world and the stomach. This makes it difficult to experience food fully in all its richness and complexity and all its pleasurable qualities.

We will describe several exercises for becoming more aware of your own mouth, for self-exploration of your oral cavity and ways to enhance its ability to sense.

Sit down in a comfortable chair and allow for fifteen to twenty minutes of privacy. Unless you have been doing the previous exercises with someone who is extremely simpatico, we suggest that you do this one alone.

Now, allow yourself to become aware of the space in your mouth. Focus on your tongue as it rests in your mouth; on the teeth as they touch each other; the molars; the front teeth. Close your eyes for a few minutes and do this again. Now concentrate on the inner space of your mouth.

Send your tongue on an exploration trip. Let it travel slowly over all of your teeth, inside and outside, deliberately, as if you were charting a map of an unknown coast. Investigate every single reef, island, inlet, ridge. Notice any difference in the texture of your teeth on the outside and the inside? How do fillings feel? What about missing spaces, sharp edges, irregularities?

Give yourself plenty of time with your teeth. It may help to close your eyes for a few minutes and repeat each portion of the trip after doing it while reading the instructions.

Then move on to the gum line at the base of your teeth. Does it feel different on the outside than on the inside? Wetter? Smoother? Cooler? Remote? Reach over beyond the last tooth, toward your distant gum. Slowly give the roof and the floor of your mouth a thorough going-over.

If you move your tongue very lightly, does it tickle? Especially toward the back of the roof of the mouth? Do you automatically make a sucking motion to stop that tickling? Can you pick out any funny or strange ridges and folds?

Now go on and feel the inside of the cheeks. Do you discern a roughness? Something like a vein in the middle of the cheek, running toward the corners of the mouth? With your tongue, push out your cheeks, one at a time.

Children like to do this — and are usually turned off with an admonition not to make funny faces.

Make a distorted face and stay in touch with how it feels. Let your tongue feel the little skin area above and below the lips in front of the teeth. Does the lower one feel like webbing? What about the upper?

Close your teeth. First, just let them rest against each other and focus on them.

Now clench them. Experience the pressure of the teeth against each other.

Center your attention on the muscles in your jaw. Feel them with your fingertips on each side, just below your ear.

TUNE IN TO THE POWERFUL PART

Relax, then clench again. Contemplate the enormous strength of these muscles.

The masseter muscle, which controls the lower jaw, is one of the most powerful in the human body. Remember the aerial artists whose clenched teeth hold a trapeze with a partner on it?

Tune in to the physical power of this part of your body. Now let your whole mouth relax. Relax your whole body for a few minutes and take a few deep breaths.

Lick your lips. Slide your tongue across the outer and inner surfaces of the lip area to the "boundary line." What texture differences come to your attention? Is the outside much rougher than the inside? Does it feel dry? Are there even tiny particles of skin that feel as if they are peeling off? Is the inside area much smoother?

Press against it hard as you move the tongue across it slowly. Is there a firm area, almost rope like?

Go to the corners of the mouth. Lick them. Is there any feeling of strangeness?

Next, let your fingertips explore your lips, following the same route as the tongue did before. What are the sensations?

Let your lips be performers. Make them tight and smooth, all the while exploring with your fingers.

Pucker them. Imagine that you are sucking a piece of lemon. How do they feel now? Form a perfect circle with your lips. Next, open your mouth as wide as you can, till you can really feel the lip tissue stretching. Touch it, with your tongue and then with your fingers. Relax for a moment or two. Take a drink of water. Now make your mouth as wide as you can. Touch the lips and then the cheeks. Do they feel unfamiliar?

Move your lips in a random fashion, making funny faces again, and keep touching them. Suck in on your lips and bite them gently. Be aware of all the tactile and kinesthetic sensations. This entire area has a wealth of nerve endings and is capable of providing many kinds of pleasurable sensations in conjunction with a wide variety of foods and beverages.

Puff out your cheeks and move the air around in them as if you were rinsing your mouth with air. Does that feel pleasant? Odd? To some people this affords a sensation never quite satisfied by eating.

Touch your puffed-out cheeks with your fingers and squeeze. Make your fingers move the air around.

Now, push your lower jaw from side to side as far as you can and let it drop as far as you can. Do you feel the joint in back? Can you hear it make sounds?

Put the end of your index finger in your mouth. Let it slowly explore your teeth the way your tongue did earlier. Usually we allow fingers to touch our teeth only in negative situations — something hurts, something is wrong, and we are trying to find out exactly what and where it is. Or maybe a tiny morsel of food is stuck between two teeth and we are trying to dislodge it.

What do your teeth feel like? The saw-like upper edge of the lower front teeth? The smooth area on the top of the molars? The point of the incisors? Many people are surprised how round the outer surfaces of their teeth feel. Others comment on the unevenness of the back teeth.

Let your fingers meet your gums. Go all around. Do you feel the invisible part of each tooth, below the gum line? Often people are amazed to find that only behind the wisdom teeth are the gums soft and spongy.

Poke around a bit more. Are you aware of salivating? Many people are unaware of the mouth as a part of the body.

Rest for a minute. How did you react to your exploration of your own mouth? Some common remarks after this exercise are: "It's like a dark cave." "I never felt all this before." "I feel evil." "I want to wash my hands; I feel uncivilized." "It's surprising what I found." "It's like wading through the primordial mud." "It's so intricate." "This is fun."

Now for a last exercise: Get a small mirror or stand in front of a mirror.

Let's closely examine a familiar part of our anatomy. Have you ever carefully looked at your mouth and inside your mouth other than to apply lipstick, or at the dentist's? Pucker your lips, then stretch them and watch the change.

Roll your lower lip over so you can see the inside. Observe how the reddish pink of the part of the lip we normally see changes to a paler pink.

Stick out your tongue. Have you ever examined your tongue (except when you have a sore throat)? Notice the irregular patterns, the ridge running clown the middle. Wiggle the tip of your tongue and become aware of its agility.

227

Next, curl your tongue up in your mouth and inspect the underside, the fine webbing. Move it back and forth like the throat of a lizard. To some people this area, under the tongue, seems like a very private and intimate area, reminiscent of the genitals.

Lastly, open your mouth wide and take a good look at the cave-like back of your throat. Say "Ah." This is another place where much sensation is experienced. Cold, sweet drinks are often quite pleasurable to this area. Focus on it. Can you feel a milkshake running down here? A cold beer on a hot day? What other beverages?

Stop now and review your feelings and thoughts during this exercise. Silly and foolish? Interesting? Peculiar? Fun?

A wide range of reactions is possible.

While "making friends with your mouth" may seem far removed from losing weight, this exercise provides you with sensitive information about your own anatomy and some heightened awareness of an area closely associated with food and eating.

15/ *HAVE A FOOD FANTASY*

We use food fantasies (sometimes called "guided day-dreams") at our workshops much as we use food awareness exercises: to help people get in touch with themselves; to find out where they are in relation to food and eating.

These fantasies are not attempts to explore a person in the psychoanalytical sense. We urge readers not to use them as a form of self-analysis. It may be interesting to conjecture whether your mother's inability to nurse you has something to do with your adult craving for hot milk with honey. But often attempts to interpret yourself get in the way of getting in touch with yourself and how you feel.

To know *where you are now* is helpful. And fantasies, like eating exercises, can aid in identifying your position now, at this moment.

In the guided fantasy it is helpful to have someone you trust read the instructions to you slowly, with many pauses. But if you are unable to have someone do this for you comfortably, we suggest you read the whole fantasy through once without trying to follow it. Then follow it from memory. Don't worry about adhering precisely to the sequence; that is quite unimportant.

To some people, the whole idea of employing a fantasy is strange and uncomfortable. If that is how you feel, we would suggest that you read the next few pages anyway. After reading further, you may find that you do want to try it. If so, just return to the beginning instructions and go ahead.

If it really turns you off, don't do it. This is not a test or hurdle that you have to pass in order to proceed. It is an experience designed to create awareness, and most people find it valuable.

Once you're ready, start the exercise. The directions follow.

HERE'S HOW

Before you attempt the fantasy, arrange for some undisturbed time in a private area — bedroom, den, study.

Allow yourself to get into a relaxed frame of mind. If this is the end of a busy day, you might have a cup of coffee or a drink first so you can feel easy and open to your imagination.

Find a comfortable position. For some people that means sprawling in a lounge chair; for others it's stretched out on a couch; for many it's lying on a soft rug on the floor. Choose whatever suits you best.

If someone is reading to you, this is where the reading starts.

●

Close your eyes and breathe deeply for a few minutes. Feel the floor for couch against your body. Notice any body tension or discomfort. Try to change that and relax more.

Now picture yourself in a meadow, lying down, enjoying the warm sun on your face. There is a sweet smell of hay and grass and the fragrance of flowers. Somewhere in the distance you can hear birds. There is a sound of running water nearby, and you can hear the wind now and then.

Spend a few minutes in this meadow. [Pause.]

Now, in your mind's eye, slowly get up. You can see a path. You follow it and find that the path leads toward the woods at the end of the meadow.

Then you notice a house at the edge of the woods. The door is slightly open. There is no one around, and you're curious to see what is inside. You open the door and walk in. You're surprised to find that inside the home are all the foods you have ever wanted to eat. It's all there and it's all yours.

There is no one else here. You can stay as long as you wish, and you can relate to the food in any way you wish.

You can stay here alone, or you can invite one or more people to join you. You can do whatever you wish — no one will disturb you. [The person doing the reading should pause here for five minutes.]

This room will always be here. You can return to it any time you wish. Whenever you feel like it, you can come back to this room full of all the food you have ever wanted.

Do whatever you please.

[Allow another pause of a few minutes.]

Now, prepare to leave in a few minutes. Remember, you can always come back.

You can linger a bit longer. See if there's anything you wish to do in the next few moments. [Pause.]

Now, walk out the door and, following the winding path, go back into the meadow.

Lie down again and rest in the grass. Let the sounds and smells of the meadow surround you. Stretch and feel the ground under you.

Now, slowly, come back into this room. Very slowly: Take several deep, slow breaths. You are back. Rest, and after a few moments sit up and open your eyes.

HOW WAS YOUR TRIP?

When you feel ready, think over your fantasy. Many find it extremely helpful to write down their "trip" — just jot down key phrases so you can examine the record any time.

How did that room look? What were the foods in it? Were any other people there? What did you do with the foods?

The instructions did not specify that you eat or not eat, only that you do whatever you wished and relate to the food. Did you eat? What foods? Did you play with them? How? Did you throw any food? How, and which ones?

How did you feel in that room? Happy? Exultant? Scared? Lonely? Guilty? Free? Invigorated? Fulfilled? Sneaky? Giddy? Awed?

What were your reactions when you were told it was time to leave soon? Did you then take time to touch more of the foods? How much did you eat? In what style? Did you hide some for another time? Were you anxious or confident? Could you picture yourself returning?

How did you feel after you left the house? Did you shut the door behind you? Lock it? Take a last-minute look? Or did you just walk away? How did you like being back in the meadow? What did it feel like to return to this room? Was this room brighter than the place in your fantasy? What are your feelings now?

The range of people's food fantasies is amazing. Earlier we described Stanley's fantasy in which he swam in chicken soup and played with huge matzo balls. This image of swimming, floating, or wading or jumping in foods occurs frequently.

Eloise, a thirty-four-year-old saleswoman, pictured herself swimming in a lake filled with meatballs and spaghetti and rich tomato sauce. As she swam, she embraced one of the meatballs (they were the size of volleyballs), and bit a chunk out of it. She flipped over on her back and floated, feeling the slippery, sensual quality of the spaghetti strands, which were four or five feet long.

The delicious smell of the sauce and garlic surrounded her totally. After a while, she became tired. She tried to move her arms, and fought harder and harder to keep from going under the surface of the sauce. But she could not help herself. She began to sink toward the bottom of the lake. At first she felt afraid. Then, she decided to let herself enjoy the warm sensations, since she couldn't do anything to save herself. To her surprise, just as she reached the bottom she felt a spongy meatball below her buttocks on the floor of the lake. The next thing she knew, there were a few more meatballs gathered underneath her body and other meatballs began to accumulate in a pyramid shape, lifting her body gradually to the surface.

As her face broke through the surface the sun was shining and she leisurely swam on her back to the shore.

You can almost anticipate what this fantasy meant to Eloise, who grew up in an Italian-American family. For years she had tried to avoid the rich dishes that were part of her background, allowing herself no lasagne, spaghetti, or fettuccini. She *tried* to avoid all high-calorie and high-carbohydrate dishes; she was terrified of becoming grossly overweight and "sinking" in her own fat, as some of her old-country relatives had. Eloise rarely ate the foods she loved. The harder she struggled with deprivation diets, the more frequent were her binges. It had become a vicious cycle and she was beginning to drown in a sea of fat — an excess of thirty-two pounds.

After the workshop, Eloise began to allow herself to eat and find pleasure in the foods that hummed to her, including many of her ethnic favorites, which she had avoided for all those years, and which had created "empty places" in her that had to be filled with other foods. As her own fantasy demonstrated, when she relaxed and enjoyed the good sensations of the foods, she began, literally, to become lighter, to "float to the surface." Her binging stopped because there no longer was a need for it. She lost twenty-eight pounds over a period of about five months, and without the agony or deprivation of dieting.

HANK'S ICE-CREAM FANTASY

Hank, a sixty-year-old minister who described himself as an ice-creamoholic, related how in his fantasy he pictured himself as a young boy. Down the center of the room was a wide conveyor belt, slowly moving. On it were huge scoops of ice cream. "Every kind of ice cream imaginable."

He had started eating, just scooping up the ice cream with his fingers and the palm of his hand as it came by. Then he kneeled over the belt and lowered his head until his mouth was right in line with the top of the scoops. Finally, he moved to the end of the conveyor belt so the ice cream simply slipped into his mouth. It was totally effortless eating at first, but gradually Hank started to feel that he, the little boy, was really being forced to eat whatever came along. He started to feel resentment at the lack of any choice, at not having an option to eat or not eat.

"The taste was still delicious, but when you said it was time to prepare to leave the room, I was glad."

Hank, who had always tried to fight his craving for ice cream, began to allow himself to eat ice cream whenever he felt like it but in a very discriminating manner. He became very particular about the exact flavor he wanted and would eat ice cream only from two specialty ice cream parlors in his city. (Previously, whenever he fell off the wagon he ate any flavor and any brand. He had often chosen the cheapest kind of ice cream in the supermarket so that he wouldn't "waste" money on his binging.) He eventually found his craving for ice cream dropping off sharply as he acknowledged and satisfied it.

Quite a different ice cream fantasy was related by Maureen, a twenty-eight-year-old nurse. When she first entered the fantasy room, she thought it was empty. "I heard the message about all the food you have ever wanted, but there was nothing in that room. I felt betrayed and lonely. But then I suddenly realized that the walls of the room themselves were made of fudge-ripple ice cream. And the pictures hanging on the walls had broad, ornate frames of crackerjack around the most fantastic layer cakes. I mean, the cakes had pictures painted on them in whipped cream and cherries and frosting.

"It was so gorgeous, I just stood there and felt happy. I finally walked up to the back wall, poked it with my finger, licked my fingers, and then licked the wall a little — so sensual! I picked a few bits and pieces off one big picture. That's all I felt like eating, which surprises me when I think back." She had expected to devour ice cream, if she ever let herself go. This was an important self-discovery. We often find that when people do let themselves go, in fantasy or in reality, they learn that their fears are unjustified; they have a lot more willpower than they had thought.

Maureen, who was twenty-four pounds overweight, had always processed food as a necessary evil. Her fantasy helped her get in touch with the fact that the esthetic appeal of food was essential to her enjoyment.

One forty-two-year-old housewife, Emily, said that when she first entered the room, it was very dim and she could hardly see anything. Gradually, as her eyes became accustomed to the subdued light, she saw that there was an enormous horseshoe-shaped buffet, "like the ones at the Vegas casinos, only even fancier than those."

She casually wandered along the table and admired all the fantastic culinary creations, from Beef Wellington with fluted mushroom caps to a salmon mousse "taller than my head," to thick crab legs resting in a bowl intricately carved out of ice, to tropical fruits arranged on a platter, like a mosaic, to "one of those marvelous French desserts. I couldn't remember the name, but it's made out of dozens of small cream puffs piled on top of each other in the shape of a tree and there is chocolate syrup all over them. This one went right up to the ceiling."

What amazed Emily was that with all this food beckoning, she never ate a bite. "I just drank two glasses of sparkling pink champagne punch."

Emily was one of the people who realized through the workshop that she had been eating nutritionally balanced meals composed of psychologically unsatisfying foods, and had been depriving herself of a range of badly needed sensations. It was not just the humming of bubbly, tart-sweet pink champagne punch, but also Coke, ice cream sodas, fruit nectars (rather than fruit juices, which was all she drank), and an occasional beer. The exclusion of so many beverages created feelings of deprivation, and she made up for them with sweet, soft desserts.

Terry, a twenty-five-year-old musician, also didn't eat much in his fantasy — until the very end. He found himself in a room full of hams, hanging salamis and bolognas, smoked beef, and other cold cuts and meats.

"I just abandoned myself to the smell of the place. It was incredibly rich and strong. I walked around sniffing, like a primitive savage. But when you said, 'Prepare to leave,' I felt panic. I started biting off chunks of salami, spitting out the skin; I stuffed chunks of thuringer into my cheeks, and I tried to grab as many things as I could. I even stuffed one huge ham down the front of my shirt."

This fantasy aided Terry, who lives in a commune, to realize how much he missed and needed unhurried eating, with time to savor the aroma and linger over the taste. Even more important, he realized that he needed to have his own, private, non-communal supply of food.

INEZ'S SWEET TOOTH WASN'T FATTENING

Inez, the twenty-nine-year-old wife of a London physician who had come to the United States on a year-long research project, had always thought that her overweight was due to her powerful sweet tooth. Her fantasy, which included diving into a room-size chocolate cake and rolling in it, helped her explore her craving for cake and chocolate. As a child in wartime England, she had been exposed to severe rationing, especially of sugar and candy, which were almost nonexistent. She had become fat after the war, and her approach to weight loss was to impose another form of rationing on herself.

Naturally, she felt compelled to break out of her diet's warlike restrictions, and binged on chocolate layer cakes, chocolate bars, etc. Through the fantasy and workshop, she realized that what she wanted most of all was a "sweet mouth," a sensation of creamy sweetness bathing her tongue and lips and mouth. Allowing the physical and sensual contact with chocolate was much more satisfying than wolfing down forbidden foods. She found she could pleasure herself with chocolate and that a small quantity of pure chocolate created a feeling of contentment for hours or even days.

Jan, a newspaper writer, sixteen pounds overweight, never ate potatoes, a childhood favorite that her grandmother used to prepare as part of every dinner. In her fantasy, she reported, as soon as she entered the room she found nothing and walked out the back door. Soon she found herself walking up a ledge trail on a rugged mountain. "I was near the summit, but there were still big cliffs towering above me. And they were all made of mashed potatoes. It was really a lovely scene, and I felt marvelous just walking along. My feet were bare and I had a delicious feeling of the mashed potatoes on my soles, and some kept squishing through my toes.

"I finally came to a long slope, like a ski run. So I sat down and slid down this gorgeous mashed-potato mountain. At the bottom there was a pool of warm potato-mushroom soup. I don't recall undressing, but when you said it was time to leave I was naked and splashing at the side of it. It didn't bother me that I was naked."

For Jan the particular combination of warm starchy potatoes with cold-warm melted butter was a sensation associated with childhood and affection. She had shunned it like the plague, but had to satisfy that loss with other foods, usually in large quantities.

Most people, as they think back over the fantasy, become aware of certain aspects of their eating and make certain connections. They notice their potential for relating to food. For guidelines, you might consider these points:

Compare the foods you enjoyed in the fantasy with the ones you pinpointed as humming foods during the food-awareness exercises. Do they coincide? If they do, this is a strong affirmation of the psychological value of such foods to you. If they don't, consider it. Were you working too hard to limit yourself in the awareness exercise and trying to stick to "healthy" (low-calorie) foods? If you didn't eat at all in the fantasy, but played with the food, explore that possibility now. Is this something you have been denying yourself? Would you like to play with food, to give yourself that experience?

Different foods have vast ranges of texture and tactile pleasure. Playing with bread or dough or chocolates are experiences normally excluded from adult behavior. In actuality they can be a rich source of sensory input. For many people food has a great deal of sensuous associations.

Let's look at another common theme. Some people in their fantasies felt like destroying the food, and actually do so. Some throw food against a wall, jump on it, or punch it. If food is still a beloved enemy to you, try to allow your anger an outlet. Go ahead: Destroy some real food. Throw it; step on it; mash it into the garbage. You may need to carry out part of your fantasy in reality before you can become more comfortable.

If your dominant feelings were anxiety, guilt, or uneasiness, you may have strong doubts about your *right* to pleasure yourself with food. Or there may be some other fear holding you back. To know how you feel is important information to have about yourself. If possible, try not to psyche yourself out by finding the explanation, though you might get some valuable insight from considering your experience in this fantasy along with the psychological exercises in later chapters.

If your feelings were mostly happy and pleasant, sensual and delightful, focus on these emotions and see how you can make the fantasy, or any portion of it, into a reality. This can become one of your passports to pleasure.

16/ *MORE EATING – AWARENESS EXERCISES*

As in the previous exercises, please do your shopping first, then arrange for some free, undisturbed time. Get a partner if there's someone you feel at ease with. If you do, have that person read the exercise to you and perhaps join you in it. If no partner is available, read through one part for directions, then reread it as you follow the instructions.

At the risk of sounding repetitive, we want to stress that this exercise, just like the others, does not contain a success-or-failure element; nor is it aimed at making you like or dislike certain foods. It is simply an aid in achieving greater food awareness, getting in touch with yourself and your sensations, and expanding the range of pleasure available from food.

Here is your shopping list;

Food Liberation Shopping List #2

✓   peanuts (dry-roasted and plain)
✓   plain milk chocolate, preferably "kisses"; otherwise, a bar that is easily broken into pre-marked sections. If possible, choose one of the thicker ones such as Swiss Tobler's or Cadbury's.

✓   1 banana

✓   plain brown paper bag, napkin

Over the years, we have encountered many people who say they are nut freaks and eat large quantities of nuts.

Nuts, of course, are thought of as chewy and crunchy, but there is a wide range of other sensations available from them. What comes to your mind when you think of nuts? What flavors, textures, sensations?

Nuts vary greatly in flavor and texture. Some are sweet, some bitter; some dry, some oily, to name just a few differences. It is worthwhile finding out which ones hum to you, in what style you eat them, and what sensation you really seek from nuts.

The Peanut Exercise

Pick up one peanut. It probably feels peculiar to pick up just one peanut, but try it anyway.

What hand is it in? Your accustomed hand? If so, change it over to the other hand. Roll it around. Now smell it. What fragrance do you pick up? Is it pungent? Some people say it reminds them of something else. Is that true with you? Any scenes come to mind? Happy? Festive? Earthy smell?

Now, run the nut across your lips and pick up all the sensations it gives you. Lips hardly ever get in contact with nuts as they are, usually, tossed into the mouth, so that lip data is missing.

Next, lick the nut. Then suck on it. Nuts are great carriers of flavor. During the usual fast eating of nuts, the surface flavor, which is largely the coating of salt, spices, and the chemical MSG, gets mixed up with the inner or true nut flavor. How do you like the coating?

Next, split the nut in half. (If it breaks into smaller pieces, discard or eat it and get a new one.) Explore the inside surface with your lips and your tongue. Notice the smoothness. Does it feel cool? Wet? What flavor, if any, do you pick up? Some people report that after contact with the pungent outer coating, the inside seems to have no flavor at all. Others detect a subtle nuttiness or a trace of an oily flavor.

Now, put one half into each side of the jaw, sliding them way back to where your gum meets your cheek, and close your mouth slowly on them. What is this like?

Run your finger along the outside of your cheek to feel the nut half. Do this on both sides, with both index fingers.

Now, with one half on each side of your mouth, take one bite. What is happening now? Do you feel a spurt of flavor? How does this compare with the flavors derived from just licking and sucking?

Once again, visualize that giant grinding up his catch. Only this time let the giant be especially strong. Put real muscle power into chewing. At the end of each chew, when your teeth are together, use your jaw muscles. Try to get in touch with all the muscles involved in your jaws and cheeks. By touching your face you can feel the jaw muscles contract. Some people can throw themselves into this to the point where they are conscious of the motion in their ear lobes, their shoulders, and the nape of the neck. This movement is meant to be slow and exaggerated, not a quick chew.

You may find that you have accidentally swallowed the nut. It is unusual to focus on one measly nut, even for an experiment. So get another nut and again put half of the nut into each side of your mouth. Chew slowly and with muscle. Now, between each chew stop to extract and suck out the flavor. Don't swallow. Continue slow chewing.

Bring the chewed-up mass forward in your mouth. Explore the texture with your tongue, then press it against the roof of the mouth, sucking at the same time to extract all possible flavor. Does this ground-nut flavor appeal to you? By now the salt and MSG flavors have all but vanished and you can evaluate the inner essence, the true nut taste.

When all flavor seems to be gone, either swallow the rest or spit it into your paper bag. Most people are surprised at how much sensory mileage can be gotten out of one nut. How was it for you?

Now, pick up another dry-roasted nut. Using mostly your front teeth, chew it as quickly as you can. Observe the sensations in your mouth. Does this nut seem different from the first one you experimented with? Do you like the blending of the coating and the inner taste? Does this seem more like "eating nuts" than the other approach? Or is it less satisfying? Swallow or spit out the nut if it hasn't disappeared already.

Repeat the same rapid-fire chewing, keeping the nut in the back of your mouth, moving your molars as quickly as possible. Again, evaluate the experience. What about the taste, the texture awareness? Check out your lips now. Do you feel they missed something, that you were cheated? Again, swallow or spit out.

How does that compare to the slow eating? People's reactions vary greatly. Some examples: "It's unfair to the nut." "I feel I'm getting cheated." "That's more like it; that's the way to eat a nut." "That really feels right, but it's funny that I don't need a whole mouthful." "I can't tell much. I need more than one nut. I need ten or twenty of them."

Do you agree with any of these, or is your position altogether different?

If you are one of the people who cannot relate to one nut, who need a whole mouthful for any real satisfaction, check yourself out on this question: Do you really crave the sensation of many nuts, or is it mostly the feeling of a full mouth that you relish?

This is not at all uncommon. In fact, that is why we put a paper napkin on your shopping list. We know that it sounds silly and peculiar to put a napkin in your mouth, but try this experiment anyway. Crumple the napkin loosely into a ball, stuff it into your mouth, and let it just sit there for a few minutes.

What's happening? Are you salivating? Does your mouth feel dry? Some people compare this to having a mouth full of cotton candy, others to being at the dentist's. Some find it revolting, some comforting; some gag, some feel they are punishing themselves, and some say it's restful.

Observe yourself. If your reactions are negative, get rid of it. If they are positive, keep it there a while. If neutral or undecided, let it remain in your mouth for a few more minutes.

We are not trying to persuade you to eat paper napkins instead of food. That would be childish and naive — even though hardly more naive than the dictates of those who rigidly count calories and would have you do pushups when you feel like eating candy, or who advocate having sex instead of eating dinner.

Again, this exercise is simply a means of gaining additional insight. Some people enjoy the sensation of having something in their mouths, and it's this sensation, rather than the taste or texture of foods such as nuts, that's important to them.

If the full-mouth feeling is a good one for you, nuts are probably inefficient in giving you satisfaction. What foods can you discover that come closer to satisfying you? Perhaps liquids that you can swish around in your mouth, or bulky foods, such as bananas. For a few people chewing gum feels good. We would like to distinguish here two different sensations: One is having a full-mouth sensation, the other is having something in your mouth to move around and play with. The latter usually requires something solid, an item that won't collapse or dissolve too quickly.

Have you ever tried a few cherry or prune pits to investigate what they might do for you? Try one. Or try several at the same time, Roll them around, let them weigh in your cheeks, rest them against the gums in back, and rub them against the gums. For some people, this can be a very pleasant experience.

A USEFUL PRUNE PIT

JoAnne, a happily married housewife and mother of three children, enjoyed cooking family meals. But she habitually tasted and snacked an extra five hundred to six hundred calories a day as she went about meal preparations. Casseroles and main dishes hummed to her, but she couldn't resist the beckoning foods around the kitchen as she cooked. For Jo-Anne a change of weight came with the insight that what she enjoyed was having something in her mouth. A prune pit proved as satisfying as her previous random picking at food. Now she can really savor family meals.

Catherine, a thirty-four-year-old real estate saleswoman from Cleveland, developed her own sophisticated version of enjoyment: She puts an unpitted olive into her after-work martini. She eats the olive as she sips and keeps the pit in her mouth while she finishes the drink.

"I roll it around and play with it with my tongue. It's a great feeling. The gin lingers on the pit. Delicious and relaxing."

Catherine was an ex-smoker. Possibly having something in her mouth satisfied some of the sensation that she missed after giving up cigarettes.

However, in the past Catherine had usually eaten a can of cocktail-mix nuts in an evening. She did not substitute the olive pits to cut down on calories. Rather, "it feels better when I have them in my mouth than the nuts ever tasted, and it feels better afterward. With the nuts, I had to chew and kept eating because I still wanted something more."

To follow up this exercise in a few days — particularly if you consider yourself a nut lover — get as many kinds of nuts as you can obtain and check them out, following the basic approach of this exercise. Even if you live in a community with limited shopping possibilities, you can pick up a can of mixed nuts and sort them out into little piles of cashews, Brazils, almonds, etc. Try to determine which kind of nut gives you the greatest pleasure and satisfaction. In the future, try to get that kind of nut. Why waste your time on second-best?

Not accepting second-best is a concept to which we keep returning because it is critically important. We have stated repeatedly that the obese person is as much entitled to the pleasures of food and eating as anyone else is. Part of this entitlement is the right to have the best — a right that many obese people deny themselves. Because they "shouldn't have candy in the first place," they will settle for a machine candy bar when they are really longing for the dark nougat from a good, old-fashioned candy shop; they will buy a package of doughy supermarket pastries when they would love a buttery Danish pastry fresh from the oven, and so on.

If you can relate to this, recall the times when you have done something like this. Was the second-best really good enough? Did it really satisfy your craving, leaving you feeling content, pleased, fulfilled rather than just full? Or were you left still craving something else?

In all probability it didn't satisfy you. It's true that it sometimes takes a little more time and energy to get the best, but the time and energy spent pleasuring yourself and meeting your need may be relatively small. (It's certainly less than what many people expend on dieting, calorie-counting, frequent weighing, and buying or preparing diet foods, not to mention the energy they need to regiment and deprive themselves!)

We mentioned that this exercise had some stopping points. We have arrived at one. If you feel you have had enough for one session, take a break now. Rest, drink, walk, think. Resume when you feel like it and when you can again arrange for free time.

The Chocolate Exercise

Unwrap one chocolate kiss (or, if you are using a thick chocolate bar, break it into squares right now).

Smell the chocolate; sniff it. At our workshops there is always a chorus of "oohs" and "ahs" when we get to this point. Smelling chocolate is a deep, sensuous delight. Yet how often do adults, even if they are self-confessed chocolate freaks, allow themselves this pleasure?

Do you usually smell chocolate before you eat it? How does it smell to you now?

(If the aroma of the chocolate alone turns you on, pick up some old-fashioned cocoa next time you're shopping. By old-fashioned, we mean the kind you have to cook, not an instant-chocolate drink. Have you ever tried cocoa? Preparing it will probably be a lovely activity for you, with the smell of chocolate pervading your whole kitchen. Drinking it is then an additional treat.)

Moisten your lips and gently rub the chocolate over them. (This, too, is something that has been educated or trained out of most of us. Children love to put chocolate on their lips, fingers, and faces, but in most households they are immediately admonished not to be messy and to eat "properly.")

How does the chocolate feel on your lips? Creamy, smooth, cool, sweet?

Now, lick your lips for the anticipatory experience of flavor, a preview, if you wish. Usually, lip-licking provides only an aftertaste. What is it like *before* the actual eating experience that will fill your whole mouth with flavor?

We realize that chocolate kisses are small, but bite off just half of one anyhow. Don't chew it, just keep it in the front of your mouth.

Allow it to stay there till it is warm enough to start to melt. Then move it into the left cheek, all the while trying not to devour it. Then move it into the right cheek. What sensations are you aware of ? "Velvety" is a word many use to describe this; others find it sticky, gooey, creamy, filling, teasing, rich. Where are you?

Try not to bite it yet, but put the piece between the front teeth and the upper lip. Slide it around with your tongue so it will coat your teeth. If there is any left, try the same with the lower teeth (or you may need a new piece anywhere along the line if the first one just vanished on you).

If there's any left, roll it around between lower lip and teeth till it's gone.

Now let your tongue follow the route of that chocolate, going back to all the places where it has been and picking up any traces that are left. Get in touch with the different sensations you experience when probing different areas. What is it like inside your cheek, between the teeth, on the gums, running your tongue along the edges of your upper or lower teeth? Are these aftersensations pleasurable?

With the next half-piece, just hold it and lick around the edges and savor the texture. Then smell again. For many, the aroma after licking is strange, but brings on pleasant mental pictures of visits to a candy store or Grandmother's cooking.

Now put it into your mouth and let it rest under the tongue so that it slowly melts there. Every so often, let the tip of the tongue check it out. How does this compare to the earlier eating?

When it is thoroughly softened, mash the chocolate against the roof of your mouth, then slide it to your favorite places, the ones where you liked your chocolate best in the first part of this exercise. With your eyes closed, get the "chocolate message." Let it dissolve totally, then rinse your mouth to clear the palate.

The next piece is not going to get the slow, tender, loving treatment. Put a whole kiss in your mouth and chew it up as fast as you can. Was that pleasant? How did it compare?

This is the way people – especially overweight people – generally eat chocolate. It is wolfed or sneaked or hustled. Yet chocolate is an inefficient food for chewing. Feelings of guilt or shame often account for the very fast demolition of chocolate. "I feel like a criminal who has to destroy all the evidence" is how one sixty-two-year-old lawyer from Baltimore put it.

While we generally don't like to make a pitch for either slow or fast eating as the "right" way, it has been our experience that very few people get deep satisfaction from chocolate unless they have time to savor it, regardless of quantity. One professed chocoholic we worked with, after slowly eating one chocolate kiss, enthused, "This has given me more pleasure than I usually get from a whole bag of chocolates that I gobble."

We suggest you repeat the whole chocolate exercise at this point and get in touch with all your feelings about it.

Instead of concentrating on pure milk chocolate flavor, all chocolate lovers can further explore their own favorites. There is a whole world of chocolate, and *you are entitled to select and eat the kind that pleases you most!* In that wonderful world of chocolate, obese people often settle for third- or fourth-best.

Many people have reported that what often hums to them is chocolate icing. Most of them will dutifully eat the cake that comes with the icing, even though they have no particular desire for cake. Typically, such persons eat several pieces of cake. They end up feeling more full than is comfortable. And they still have not had as much icing as they had craved.

If you really love the icing totally by itself, make a batch of icing, or buy a can of it, and eat it with a spoon. (We've never enjoyed the canned icing, personally.) If you like a minor taste of cake with your hardened icing (as the majority seems to want), ask the bakery to cut out the soft center of the cake, or do it yourself at home if you're too embarrassed to ask in public. If you bake yourself, try baking one thin layer of cake and then ice it thickly. Or check out how you like thin butter cookies, or even graham crackers, thickly spread with icing.

A favorite in many teen-age summer camps is "somemores," an exotic and gooey concoction of a graham cracker (as a base), half a plain Hershey chocolate bar, toasted marshmallows, and another graham cracker to cap it off. The warm marshmallows melt some of the chocolate, which is then absorbed by the cracker. Try it — it's an unusual blend of sweet tastes.

One woman who came to a New York workshop invented what she called her super-treat: a sandwich made of several imported Petit Beurre cookies with thick layers of chocolate icing in between.

This relates to an earlier point: the enslavement to rules that dictate *how* something should be eaten and *when* it should be eaten. There is no reason why chocolate icing can be eaten only on a slice of cake. Nor is there any reason why chocolate, in whatever form you like, can be considered as only a dessert or treat.

In Mexican cooking, chocolate is used in sauces for meat (*molé*); for many German children, hot chocolate is the customary breakfast drink; and in Holland, a regular breakfast feature is bread and butter with "Hundreds and Thousands," which are small chocolate morsels.

Anthelme Brillat-Savarin (1755-1826), the noted French politician and gastronome, wrote: "Chocolate is one of the most effective restoratives. All those who have to work when they might be sleeping, men of wit who feel temporarily deprived of their intellectual powers, those who find the weather oppressive, time dragging, the atmosphere depressing; those who are tormented by some preoccupation which deprives them of the liberty of thought; let all such men imbibe a half-litre of *chocolat ambré* [a chocolate with a musk-like odor which was then popular in France] and they will be amazed."[*]

Hot chocolate is, of course, a very satisfying drink for people who like chocolate and who want warmth at the same time as sweetness. Check yourself out on this. At what temperature is chocolate most "chocolatey" to you? For some people the greatest enjoyment is coupled with warmth (hot chocolate, hot fudge, chocolate fondue). For others the opposite is true (chocolate ice cream, chocolate milkshakes, Eskimo pies.)

Texture or consistency is important, too. Full realization of pleasure often hinges on fine nuances.

A doctor we worked with in a weekend group remembered that one of the best childhood treats *for him* had been licking the pot after his mother had made chocolate pudding. He often ate chocolate pudding and found it pleasant, but not as good as that pot-licking experience way back then. He finally found the answer when his young daughter cooked some pudding for Daddy as a special birthday treat and got lumps in it: He loved the lumps! There had always been small lumps and areas near the top of the pot where the pudding was hardened and not as smooth as pudding "should be."

For others, chocolate should be hard. Broken milk-chocolate chunks are often favorites with them. For still others the chocolate is enhanced by the addition of something chewy, like nuts or caramel.

---

[*] Cited in Prosper Montagne*Larousse Gastronornique* (New York: Crown, 1961).

At a Reno workshop, there was a mid-fortyish woman who ran a neighborhood dry cleaning shop. For years she had eaten large quantities of Hershey bars, always feeling guilty and never getting full satisfaction from them — although they did taste good. The food-awareness exercises brought her in touch with the fact that the bars lacked several qualities which were essential to her being able to find lasting pleasure in chocolate: The chocolate had to be creamy, sweet, and cold.

She experimented with chilled "hot chocolate," chocolate creams well refrigerated, chocolate ice cream sodas and shakes. All of these she found pleasant. But what she described as her "ultimate chocolate experience" was Kahlua (the Mexican liqueur) with milk over ice.

She was startled when someone pointed out that Kahlua is actually a sweet coffee liqueur. But this discovery didn't faze her. "I don't care if it is. To me it's chocolatey, brown, and sweet, and it's perfect."

Other chocolate freaks reported their surprised happiness when they were turned on by some of the genuine chocolate liqueurs, such as Vandermint (a minted chocolate liqueur from Holland), crème de cacao, and Swiss chocolate liqueur. *Capucchino*, the steaming Italian hot chocolate with brandy, can be satisfying for those craving warm sweetness.

None of these examples may apply to you. You might find semisweet chocolate bits exciting, or chocolate Ovaltine, or Heath bars, or Cadbury's chocolate-covered shortbread, or Toblerone, or chocolate-flavored yoghurt. When or if chocolate hums to you, we urge you to give yourself a complete chocolate checkup. Investigate and explore the wide, wide world of chocolate, the total range of textures, qualities, aromas, tastes

257

available in chocolate. And then make sure you get exactly what you want! The best box of candy will literally leave something to be desired if hot fudge is humming to you. And the thickest, creamiest double-chocolate shake cannot fill the void left by the unmet craving for a bag of M&Ms.

Once again, we are at a good stopping point, a good place to take a break before we proceed with the banana.

Even if you are eager to go on, we suggest a cup of coffee or a drink of milk or water to clear the palate, and a few minutes to contemplate what you've just experienced and discovered about yourself.

The Banana Exercise

Bananas are a sadly misunderstood and neglected food. The calorie-counters condemn them because they are high in calories. Others consider them something for kids, or a substitute for meals, since many diet schemes say bananas are taboo except when eaten in place of lunch or dinner.

However, let's explore the taste and texture of a banana, both of which are unique to it.

Peel your banana; break it in half, then break off a one--inch piece. Do you realize that the growth pattern of bananas is such that you can easily break a piece of banana into thirds? It splits from its core into three almost equal sections. Try it.

Observe the difference of texture on the outside and inside surfaces. Explore it with your tongue.

Now smell the banana and absorb the aroma slowly and deliberately. Many people are surprised here. As one woman put it, "I always thought bananas smelled blah, but they don't. It's really an unusual and interesting smell." How does it smell to you? Pleasant? Unpleasant?

Hold the piece of banana in your unaccustomed hand — have you became used to doing that by now? — and bring it up to your lips. Then slide it into your mouth. Don't bite or chew the banana yet.

Mash it against the roof of your mouth and squeeze hard with your tongue as if you were a juice extractor. What is the sensation? Is your main reaction "sweet," or do you pick up other components? Does the taste resemble the smell? Is there an oiliness, a touch of bitterness in the sweetness or a milky quality?

Move the pulp around, letting it glide along the teeth, both upper and lower, inside and out, and keep yourself open to the differing experiences, the nuances of flavor, and occasionally the absence of flavor. Let the flavor fill your mouth before swallowing.

Savor the aftertaste. What elements are dominant? Is there still a remnant of the aroma you noticed first, before tasting?

Many of the essential qualities of a banana are wasted when the fruit is chewed. Consider the fact that your teeth played a totally passive role in the eating of that small piece of banana. You only ran the pulp along the teeth and against the roof of your mouth. Yet most people find that they experience unsuspected and definite flavors in this exercise. Did you?

Bananas are unlikely to appeal much to those who crave a chewing experience, but they are superbly suited to those

259

who like to mash and "squoosh" their food. Children are sometimes criticized for having a "lazy mouth" when they don't chew vigorously. This can happen because the child is mashing and pureeing food. And that is a perfectly legitimate way of eating for some people, a way of obtaining pleasure from food.

Pick up another piece of banana. (Which hand is it in?) Now, with your tongue, explore the textures once more — the fibrous and rough outside, the smooth, slippery inside, and then, once again, the harder inner core.

Now put a piece into either cheek against the lower gum line. Bring the palm of your hand up against the outside of your jaw and mash the banana with the pressure from your hand only. Get in touch with all of your sensations: the tactile experience of both outer and inner cheek surfaces, the gums and hand, plus the taste experience as flavor is released.

When the banana is very soft, start running it through your teeth slowly.

Is that appealing or disagreeable? Many people find it soothing, "like rinsing your mouth with a pleasant, warm liquid." Let this process last as short or as long a time as you please.

On the next piece, using your front teeth and holding the banana in your fingers, scrape off the rough outside. You now have the slick, smooth inner surface totally exposed, which is different from the way you usually know a banana.

Bring the piece up to your lips. Let it glide over your lips. Now explore it with your tongue. Is this pleasurable?

Put it in your mouth and move it around there, exploring it all the while.

Now, in a complete change of pace, break off a piece of banana and chew it up very rapidly.

What's your reaction? Was this more "normal," or did it feel strange, out of place?

Evaluate the taste experiences you gained from the first, slow style of eating and from this fast chewing method. Does banana appeal to you as a chewing food, or more for gumming and mashing, or not at all? Some people do like to chew a banana, even though it is too soft for real sink-your -teeth-into-it chewing. But it has staying power and doesn't collapse or vanish on you (like much softer foods, such as ice cream and puddings).

Many people who desire a full-mouth feeling find bananas highly satisfactory. So do people who cherish a delicate aftertaste that lingers long after the eating activity has ceased. Others, even some who have been eating bananas for many years, frequently find that, after experimenting, they really don't like bananas, that they are "too mild and dull" or "neither a food nor a drink" or "a sweet that isn't sweet enough."

(Incidentally, the foods that you didn't eat can be saved for further exercises; or to be eaten when they hum; or you can throw away whatever you don't want.)

A vast underworld of sensations is available in bananas and all other foods. Start exploring now, experimenting and discovering the world of food. You can embark on your own exploration any time. Reexamine familiar foods and investigate new ones solely in terms of the sensory qualities that food can offer you according to your mood and cravings.

This is part of the way to liberated eating and permanent weight loss. The more satisfaction and pleasure you have in eating, the less need there is for excessive eating or for overeating.

Part III

FREQUENTLY ASKED QUESTIONS — AND
THE ANSWERS

17/ *FREQUENTLY ASKED QUESTIONS*

What About Medical Advice on Dieting?

Question: I have borderline diabetes and should not eat any sweets at all. But your method encourages me to ignore medical advice.

Answer: No. At no time do we encourage anyone to ignore their physician's advice. Our concern is with freeing people from food hang-ups and battles, so they can eat *in a natural manner* even if they must live with a food handicap because certain foods are medically out of bounds. Such a handicap, too, is part of your natural being We've worked successfully with people who had severe diabetes, hypercholesterolemia, ulcers, etc., and were supposed to watch sweets, fats, or other foods. But these people were obese and were eating food they knew they shouldn't. They were unable to heed the medical warnings or cautions they had been given. In other words, knowing what not to eat does not automatically bring about a change in eating behavior. If people were able to follow medical advice (assuming it was something they believed and accepted) we would not have any smokers, alco-

holics, overeaters, or obese people in this country. Information alone is not sufficient to change
emotionally loaded areas of human behavior.
Our method helps people to use their doctor's
advice, not to ignore it.

Women Have Special Problems

Question: Why do so many of my women friends spend so
              much time overeating and then trying to lose
              weight?

Answer: In our society women are trained to put the
              needs of others before their own. If a woman is
              always giving to others, she must find some way
              to give to herself or become emotionally de-
              pleted. Often the only channel left for giving to
              oneself is through food. Also, as we discussed in
              this book, women have been taught to view
              themselves as objects that are more desirable if
              they have a "perfect figure." The whole cycle of
              dieting, guilt, deprivation (and overeating) oc-
              curs in order to achieve that goal.

Can Food Fight Loneliness?

Question: I am divorced and I think I overeat to compen-
              sate for my loneliness. How can I stop eating
              cookies and cake when I feel lonely?

Answer: Your question sounds like: "What do I do about
              feeling so lonely?" We assume that if you could

arrange your life differently, you would not be alone, so any suggestions about finding companionship would be insulting.

One way to deal with loneliness is to experience it fully. There are solid reasons why you are lonely, and loneliness is a powerful emotion. Trying to ignore it or suppress it or deny it makes no sense and is usually unsuccessful. For many, loneliness is a fact of reality, of existential sadness, and part of living. It may even be helpful to admit or acknowledge that your loneliness is a sad and painful experience, and may be worth crying about.

When someone feels lonely or hurt or emotionally battered by life, she deserves comforting and tenderness, even if self-administered: a warm bath with your favorite bath oil, or buying some flowers (or even sending half a dozen roses to yourself) or a massage or appointment at the hairdresser — whatever you enjoy for comforting yourself.

Finally, eating chocolate or cookies or candy or cake may be extremely soothing and comforting for loneliness — perhaps eating finger foods all evening instead of a regular dinner can be a pleasant experience. In other words, allow the cookies and cake to be effective soothers, rather than try to omit the very things that assist you in coping with the world.

What's Unique about Liberated Eating?

Question: What do you think are the most important fea-
              tures of your program that distinguish it from
              others?

Answer: You eat the foods you love; you free yourself
              from guilt; you use Eating-Awareness Exercises
              and fantasies to learn about your "hunger"; you
              stop battling yourself with diets. With freedom
              from guilt and dieting comes freedom from the
              compulsion to overeat. You no longer have to
              stuff yourself today for fear that tomorrow you
              will really have to put yourself on that impossi-
              bly strict diet. You break the vicious cycle. In
              the old days you thought you would have to be
              on such a diet forever. Without this dreaded
              possibility, there is no need for guilt-ridden
              gorging and hinging.

What to Do about Late-Night Eating

Question: I teach school. My children usually go to bed at
              9:00 P.M. I look forward to my time alone, but
              from about 10:00 P.M. on, I seem to eat nonstop
              until I finally go to sleep around midnight.
              Nothing hums to me and yet I have a real hun-
              ger of some kind.

Answer: There is the possibility that you may be using
              food as a way of procrastinating, as a way of
              seizing extra time instead of going to bed. Peo-

ple who eat late at night often feel cheated of *time*. They use food in order to stay awake. The food doesn't give quick energy, but it gives bursts of sensation that can stimulate whoever is trying to stay awake (or drive for a while or run lots of errands).

Why resist going to bed earlier? For some people it means being cheated of solitude and time alone without children, demands, and discussion. In that case you have to decide what you really want to do about your time. If you decide you can't give up that evening time, experiment with distinct, strong-tasting snacks. Also, could dinner be postponed for that needy period between 10:00 P.M. and midnight?

People who force themselves to stay up late at night, ignoring body demands for sleep, sometimes do this because of a problem about their self-concept. Inside, their thinking goes something like this: "All the beautiful people, the jet-setters, the people who live exciting, romantic, productive lives, stay up late; going to bed early is almost a condemnation or proof of my living an uneventful and dull life."

We encourage people to follow their body signals, including going to bed when they're tired. Using food to capture time at night is inefficient. If you need time alone without children, for example (as most mothers do) you might try to arrange for some such time during the day. The wish to live a more exciting life can be realized in other, more direct ways. An evening at home can be enjoyably spent with hobbies or even outright loafing!

Will a Substitute Do?

Question: My great passion is Three Musketeers candy bars. Some candy machines at work don't have those. Is it all right to get some other candy or is it important that I get Three Musketeers?

Answer: It is important to satisfy your taste preferences precisely. A substitute candy, even if similar, may leave you feeling not quite satisfied and still hungry.

Controlling Children's Eating of Sweets

Question: I can see the value of liberated eating for myself, but I would still like to control my children, aged six, eight, and eleven, and what they eat. I feel that such young children need my guidance for healthy and nutritious eating.

Answer: Children eventually have to take responsibility for their choices, including what they eat. First of all, policing how and what and when your children eat simply doesn't work. We recall working with one teen-age girl whose parents tried to control her eating. Her response was not only to sneak food at school, but eventually she started waking up in the middle of the night so that she could have something to eat in peace. This household became almost unbelievably tense. When the father and mother found out about this midnight marauding they started taking turns staying up all night so they could help their daughter "control her night eating." The mother would say to her daughter, "Don't you know what you're doing? Every bite you take is killing you, and look what you're doing to me!" At first the girl had had one peanut-butter sandwich every night. With her mother or father "helping" she felt compelled to eat three or four.

A number of mothers who, after attending our workshop, stopped policing their children and instilling them with guilt about eating, reported that the children showed dramatic weight loss and eventually nutritionally better eating. Parental patience during the adjustment period is helpful.

Eating to Quell a Bad Taste in the Mouth

Question: Sometimes I have a bad taste in my mouth and look for something to eat that will make me feel better. Any suggestions?

Answer: Try brushing your teeth or using a mouthwash. *Then* explore whether there is still anything you want to eat.

What about WW, TOPS, and OA?

Question;   You criticize Weight Watchers, TOPS, and simi-
            lar organizations. Don't those groups do any-
            thing valuable?

Answer: Yes, they do. The need for such groups grew out
            of the fact that the traditional medical approach
            was largely unsuccessful. One of the pioneers in
            the field, TOPS, organized nearly twenty-five
            years ago, provided desperately needed emo-
            tional support for people with weight problems.
            The proliferation of such organizations today —
            including not only WW and TOPS, but Lean
            Line, Calories Anonymous, Overeaters Anon-
            ymous, Dieters of America, Weight Off With
            Sense (WOWS), and many more — attests to
            the continuing need for approaches other than
            the medical. The need for new methods is also
            shown by the recent survey of the success of
            dieting and pills under medical supervision, as
            reported by Dr. Samuel Waxier of the University
            of California Medical School in San Francisco.
            Follow-up studies showed a 98 percent failure to
            maintain weight loss; there was only a 3 percent
            success rate.

            Our primary objection to the methods used
            by almost all diet organizations is the stress on
            control, discipline, willpower, and other out-
            moded psychological concepts. We feel that
            such an approach contributes to feelings of fail-

ure, inadequacies, guilt, and other dysfunctional feelings.

Still, some people benefit from those methods, at least for a while. If you can feel comfortable with their way of relating to food, that's fine with us. Do whatever works for *you*.

Trapped in the Kitchen

Question.   I don't like cooking very much and resent having to spend a lot of time in the kitchen, but my family enjoys good food and being together at mealtime. I feel trapped.

Answer: Here are a few possibilities:

•   Everybody in the family can pitch in and help with the daily preparation of meals.

•   Keep dinners very informal, mostly buffet-style. And don't hesitate to make use of the multitude of convenience foods now available. There is no reason to feel guilty or negligent about using these, rather than cooking from scratch.

•   It may not be practical and economical to do this often, but it's fun and very liberating: Enjoy time together while you drive around getting each family member exactly what hums to him or her. That might mean a stop at the pizza parlor, a visit to McDonald's, picking up some Chinese food "to go," or even getting a certain TV dinner at the supermarket.

Pleasure Chart for a Bread Freak

Question: I'm a bread freak from way back. I'm ecstatic
that you've helped me feel it's all right to eat
bread. Any suggestions about how I could pleasure myself with bread even more?

Answer: Try different ways of eating; make up your own
bread-awareness exercises after the pattern of
food-awareness exercises in the book. You might
eat only the crust or only the inside. Roll some
of the bread into a ball, then smell the yeasty
aroma that clings to your hands; gum this bread
ball, etc.

Another experience that has been described
as unusually sensuous is this: Take a whole loaf
of French bread and cut it in half. Hollow out
one half by taking out the bread with your fingers. When it's hollow, and has just the outer
shell of crust, put your hand into it for a few
minutes. Feel the wall and coolness.

Now, take your hand out and bring the bread
shell to your face, like a mask. Smell the bread
aroma, the coolness, and the dough almost sur-
rounding you. It's a total bread experience.

Also, you can explore a wide range of breads.
Buy as many different kinds as you can find and
see which ones are satisfying.

Ideally, a bread experience involves not only
taste and touch but smell, especially the smell
of bread baking. This you can enjoy without

starting from scratch, what with all sorts of breads and rolls available frozen and ready for you to bake.

If you are ambitious, the process of real bread-baking can yield all sorts of pleasurable sensations: Feeling the flour, having the warm dough stick to your hands in the original mixing of ingredients; later, the highly satisfying continuous motion of kneading; the slapping of the dough on the board. Yeast is marvelous to smell and to watch in action — the rising of yeast bread is a living process. When you make yourself part of this process, it is easy to understand why, along with wine, bread ("the staff of life") is the foodstuff to which most symbolism is attached.

"I Can't Eat at My Own Dinner Parties"

Question: When I give a dinner party I have a hard time enjoying the food, even if I serve something that had been humming to me and looks delicious.

Answer: It might be a good idea for you to postpone eating until after your guests leave. Socializing and eating don't mix for many people. Personally when I (Lil Pearson) give a dinner party, I don't eat until it's over. I find it easy to postpone eating, waiting for when it will be pleasurable. I used to find that when I ate during my dinner parties, I still felt hungry after the guests left, so I'd wind up eating again. This doesn't happen anymore.

Vomiting to Lose Weight

Question: I'm ashamed to ask about this. I vomit after some meals, almost daily. I don't mean that I have to vomit. I make myself vomit.

Answer: About 10 percent of our workshop participants use vomiting as a means of weight control. Of all the topics discussed in our groups — use of pills, fasting, hormone shots, enemas — self-induced vomiting seems to be the most difficult to discuss with others. Most vomiters feel acute shame, yet are relieved when they find out they are not the only ones who engage in this practice. They usually do it because overeating and nervousness make food "sit like a brick."

Mary Ellen, a fairly slender woman, wife of an architect and mother of four children (ages five, seven, eight, and eleven) told how she feared that her children might discover that she often made herself vomit. ("It's usually after dinner, when I feel stupid and all choked up and hate myself for having eaten too much.") When she made herself vomit she felt this was a shameful practice, "worse than being caught masturbating."

Mary Ellen's problem was that she wasn't sufficiently selective about when, where, how, and what she ate. After our basic workshop she realized that most of the time she did *not* enjoy eating with her children and she viewed this feeling as unnatural. She enjoyed eating alone or having a quiet dinner with just her husband. When *everything* hummed to her — the food, the place, the people, and the time — she enjoyed her food, didn't overeat, and felt no need to vomit.

Many mothers of young children find it upsetting to eat with children who are messy, sloppy, unaesthetic, and demanding of mother's energy. Rather than calling this non-maternal or pathological, we believe this is a normal reaction for some people. We encourage these mothers to keep their children company, but to eat separately.

While vomiting is perhaps the least socially acceptable "solution" to overeating, in the long run it is no more damaging than appetite-suppressant pills or enemas.

Is Overeating an Illness?

Question: My friend from Overeaters Anonymous says overeating is an illness. What do you think?

Answer: We totally disagree. As the name implies, Overeaters Anonymous utilizes the Alcoholics

Anonymous approach with food. The assumption is that overeating is a physiological addiction comparable to alcohol or drug addiction. There is no scientific evidence to support this. In fact, all scientific evidence speaks against this theory.

"How Can I Control My Chocolate Consumption?"

Question: My main weakness is eating chocolate, lots of it, and I hate myself for it. It often has nothing to do with being hungry. What can I do to stop eating chocolate?

Answer: Nothing. So long as the issue is phrased in this kind of archaic language, no answers are possible in the language of liberated eating — or probably any other language.

The issue is: Can you accept the need for chocolate and learn how to intensify the pleasure and satisfaction you derive from it? In a recent workshop, a salesman described himself as devouring chocolate when he was nervous. During the workshop it became apparent that he rarely experienced the chocolate. He found that when he allowed himself the valid use of chocolate and then explored it to the maximum — letting it melt under his tongue, mashing it against the roof of his mouth, etc. — he gained a much more intense pleasure. Subsequently, less chocolate was necessary to provide more satisfaction.

Transition Eating between Errands

Question: I eat a lot during the day, snacking while rushing around on errands and jobs. Any suggestions?

Answer: It's valuable to check out whether you are using food as a transition activity. This kind of eating serves as a bridge between one activity and another, such as coming home from the office and fixing dinner, or between two errands, or while driving.

At these times people may really crave a nap, a hot bubble bath, or other body comfort, yet they turn to food as a substitute. This tends to leave the original craving unsatisfied. It may be helpful to experiment with alternate ways of achieving body comfort. You may find that the transition between two worlds or two chores is most efficiently dealt with by lying down for a few minutes between activities or by allowing time for a hot bath or shower.

All body comfort needs (as well as emotional needs) are valid. It is very important to accept this concept and then to satisfy the needs in the most efficient manner possible.

Transition eating is necessarily almost always hurried. Bland, non-distinctive foods tend to get lost in this shuffle. They are processed but not experienced and therefore are not very satisfying. For most people, something with a dominant, unique, or powerful taste, which just cannot be ignored, is a good choice. So are very hot or very cold foods.

Check yourself out on this, and if it is food or beverages that you want, make sure that it's always handy. My (Lil's) favorite transition foods are raw zucchini, sliced thin, with salt and spicy herbal French salad dressing. It takes only one or two minutes to prepare; you can make a batch and leave it on the counter all day or in the refrigerator if you like it chilled. It's crunchy and spicy.

Do the New Body Therapies Help Lose Weight?

Question: What about the new "body therapies," such as Primal therapy, Gestalt therapy, bioenergetics, Rolfing, polarity therapy, etc.?

Answer: We feel that these new methods of developing human potential have much to offer and have known people who benefitted from these approaches. Unfortunately, these methods seem to have little to offer regarding weight loss. In our workshops we have frequently had people who have been through a variety of the newer body therapies. They feel better about some aspects of their lives, and are more in touch with their bodies, but haven't achieved subsequent change in weight or eating patterns.

Obsession with Forbidden Food

Question: The minute I decide   *not* to have something,
              then I get obsessed with wanting it.

Answer: This is precisely why diets don't work in the
              long run. Depriving oneself has limits beyond
              which a person won't go! What you say reminds
              me (Lil) of a recent episode. I went to my bro-
              ther's birthday party on a Sunday afternoon. I
              had decided beforehand that I wouldn't have
              any alcoholic drinks, not because of dieting, but
              because later in the afternoon I would have to
              be driving my children for quite a distance.
              When we got to the party there was a gigantic
              crystal bowl full of martinis with a huge cake of
              ice floating in the middle and olives marinating
              right in the bowl. Sticking to my resolve I got
              myself a glass of water and kept reminding my-
              self that I usually don't like drinking in the
              afternoon anyhow. But watching all those other
              people drinking, and having forbidden it to
              myself beforehand, I started feeling more and
              more deprived. Finally, I left the party and
              drove my children to their appointment. When I
              came back to the party I eagerly rushed for the
              martini bowl. I even got myself a real glass rath-
              er than one of the plastic glasses that were being
              used.

                  Almost with trembling hands I ladled up the
              martini and eagerly sipped it — only to be

shocked! It didn't taste good! I hadn't truly wanted it at all, but I had made it into forbidden fruit and thereby lost perspective on what I was feeling.

Do You Always Eat Only Foods That Hum?

Question: Are *you* (the Pearsons) always able to limit your eating to just foods that hum?

Answer: No. Let me describe what recently happened to me (Len). I came home late from campus. It had been a tiring day. The weather was cold, damp, and foggy. On the way back home I pictured hot, thick, steaming split-pea soup with potatoes and rice. As I opened the door, the pungent aroma of garlic bread flooded over me. This is one of my favorite foods.

    My daughter Andrea proudly announced that since Lil wasn't feeling well, she had taken over responsibility for cooking dinner and was just about finished with a delicious meat-cheese-noodle casserole, which is also one of my favorites. She was proud of her efforts, and I promptly forgot my "soup message."

    After eating the casserole, a small green salad with crumbled Roquefort cheese, and the garlic bread, I wanted a taste of something cold and sweet and had a few spoons of chocolate-swirl ice cream, "for dessert." About an hour later I felt myself craving more ice cream. I ate some more. About a half hour later I yearned for still more. After eating over half a quart and feeling absolutely stuffed, I knew something was wrong. I searched back over the afternoon and evening and realized that I was rewarding myself for having been deprived of that humming split-pea soup. At this point I didn't feel any further craving for ice cream.

During the next day, I still felt full from the previous night's dinner and had only a cup of tea for breakfast and also for lunch.

This was another foggy, damp day on campus and before leaving for the hour's drive, I phoned ahead to make sure that there would be some split-pea soup simmering by the time I got home. It was. And that's all I felt like eating.

Candy and Quick Energy

Question: I'm holding down two jobs to make ends meet and often I'm really worn out. That's when I eat candy, to give myself some quick energy. Is that all right?

Answer.   Sure it's all right, but not because it gives you quick energy. The myth that candy or other sweets will provide you with instant energy seems to die hard. Even pure sugar does not get metabolized and become available for about twenty minutes. With most candies the process takes longer.

If you feel an immediate pickup when you eat candy (and many people do) it is because of the stimulus provided by the sweet sensation in your mouth or throat. This is a valuable experience, and eating candy for that purpose, at times when you feel in need of a boost, is a legitimate use of food. But be sure to get the candy that provides you with the most eating pleasure.

The Danger of Surrendering to Food

Question: I'm eating all the food I like most of the day, and I'm gaining weight. How do you explain that?

Answer: It sounds as if you are surrendering to food, rather than taking time and effort to find out what hums to you and to develop awareness or food sensitivity.

We read a story in the newspaper recently about a couple who had been poor all their lives. Suddenly they won a large sum of money. They immediately went on an incredible buying binge and, within a few months, blew the whole bundle. Then they returned to their old lifestyle. It was as if they couldn't stand having that much wealth; as if they were sure someone would take it away from them, or that they simply didn't believe they deserved it in the first place.

You're eating the foods you like "most of the day," and that sounds similar to that couple.

Being centered on yourself, on what hums to you, and being sensitive to food can require effort. It can be a lot of work — especially at the beginning. What's most important is that you have to allow yourself time for the new learning to take place so you can discriminate between foods and your authentic reactions to them.

What's Wrong with a Reward?

Question: Why is it wrong to reward a child with ice cream when he has eaten all his dinner?

Answer: That's not a reward, that's a bribe. Such deals are invariably conditional. It's "*If* you eat all your dinner like a good boy, *then* I'll give you the ice cream." By doing this, you are also elevating ice cream to a super special position. You are saying that it is really more desirable than any of the rest of the meal. Instead of helping the child tune in to himself, you are conditioning him to view ice cream as a special food, not just a taste experience about which he can make up his own mind.

Finding the Optimal Combination of Foods

Question: I understand what liberated eating means, but I have a special problem. At times I crave a combination of tastes that aren't available in any one food. For example, sometimes I want something with the following qualities: soft, chewy, sweet, doughy, crunchy, and something I can eat with my hands.

Answer: When no food seems to exist that would satisfy a set of sensations you crave, you need to experiment and create your own.

One recipe that combines the above qualities follows:

Oatmeal Chews

Cream: 1 c. sugar
1 egg
¼ c. milk
4 tsp. molasses
1 tsp. vanilla

Add: 1 c. melted butter
1 ¾ c. flour
2 c. oats
1 tsp. cinnamon
½ c. sunflower seeds
¾ c. chopped walnuts
¾ c. raisins
½ tsp. salt
1 tsp. baking powder.

Drop onto cookie sheet by the teaspoonful. Bake at 350° for fifteen minutes.

Explore other combinations and see what works for you. There are many ways of baking your own bread with exotic ingredients. Try some of those, but don't feel bound by an exact recipe. Reconsider all the recipe books you have in terms of "What *sensations* and *textures* can I find, as well as taste qualities?" So far as we know, no recipe book exists with chapter headings such as: "Sweet, brittle foods," "Cold, tart, chewy dishes," "Warm, sweet, crunchy snacks," "Soft, hot, carbohydrate/dough/starch flavor treats." But you can search out the tastes you want from your old stand-by cookbooks.

When a Child Worries Over Mother's Weight Loss

Question: My six-year-old daughter keeps saying I'm too skinny now. How can I convince her that she was simply used to seeing me fat? I don't want to hurt her feelings.

Answer: Children often feel insecure and need reassurance when a dramatic change of any sort occurs with a parent. When one aspect of the parent changes — like Mother losing weight — the child wonders, "What else might change? How about her love for me?" Children usually are not conscious of this reasoning. Verbal reassurance is effective. If you can, spend a little extra time with your daughter. You might let her come along when you shop for new clothes or prepare some of your favorite foods together.

"How Can I Stop Eating All the Courses at Dinner?"

Question: I understand and follow liberated eating, and usually eat only foods that hum. But at a restaurant or a dinner party I seem to want some of everything — even if it's something I don't especially like. I eat the appetizer, salad, soup, bread, main dish, vegetables, and dessert, although soup and salad hardly even beckon to me — ever! What's going on with me?

Answer: Perhaps the completeness (totality) of a meal is what hums to you. Many dieters, especially those who have been living deprived lives since childhood, vividly recall times when they ate "incomplete" (or, as one workshop member put it, "amputated") meals. Her mother always removed the potatoes from her dish, gave her no butter and only one half slice of bread and half portions of dessert (if any), except on such special occasions as birthdays. She did not know what it meant to eat a whole meal until she started living away from home at college.

You may be responding to the normal feeling of being able to have all the courses without any crippled portions or amputated servings. Perhaps you need to allow yourself this experience for a while before you no longer need to treat yourself.

Another possibility may have to do with being served and waited on. To some people this is so pleasurable that it seemingly makes everything hum. But only seemingly. Check it out.

Self-Rewarding Is O.K.

Question: I'm a college student and always fill up on candies and chocolate bars when I'm studying for an exam. I know I'm rewarding myself in advance, but it seems like a dumb thing to do because getting a high grade on the test should be enough of a reward.

Answer: The distress that's associated with studying for an exam is a frequent and logical experience. Making up for this distress in the present, by means of a reward, particularly sweet foods, makes good psychological sense. The notion of attaining your reward at some future date through a high grade is an example of trying to use abstract and future events to deal with present needs. In our experience, once you can acknowledge that eating chocolate prior to an exam is valid and legitimate, the amount of chocolate needed to do its work becomes smaller.

Pre-Menstrual Tension and Eating

Question: I can't seem to control my eating just before my period and I know that I have pre-menstrual tension. What can I do so that I don't eat so much?

Answer: This is very common. Many women describe their craving for chocolates and sweets prior to their period. Some authorities feel there may be a biochemical basis for this. Others believe it has a psychological cause, with the woman emotionally preparing herself for the impending loss of body fluids. Another explanation is that there is a need to reward oneself in advance for the stress sometimes associated with menstruation.

To deal with this in a liberated way, evaluate what sensations you are seeking, what would be most comforting to you. In some cases it may be sweets. If so, select the kind that pleases you most. You may find other rewarding activities. Try to explore other ways to treat yourself each month. You are entitled to it.

The "Best" Chocolate

Question: Can you tell me which brand of chocolate is best?

Answer: We can't. The best chocolate is the one *you* like best. We use certain foods in our workshops —

and recommend them for eating exercises in our book — only because they come in convenient units.

"I Can't Stop Myself"

Question: Once I begin to eat a meal, especially dinner, I eat until I'm stuffed. I just can't seem to stop myself. I don't even know when I'm full, except when all the dishes are empty. What can I do?

Answer: Try a "mid-meal meander." Because of the competing stimuli at dinnertime — companions, reading, TV, food aromas, beverage tastes, etc. — it may be difficult to become aware of the sensation of feeling full. We suggest you stand up periodically and walk away from the dining area. Go to another room, look out of a window, or sit in an easy chair. Look upon this *not* as a way of making yourself stop eating, but rather as a way of examining where you are. This gives you an opportunity to observe your own sensations and a chance to make a conscious *decision* about what you wish to do.

"I'm Still Worried"

Question: Generally, I feel good and free about my eating now, but I still have my old silly fear that my

Answer:

favorite food might disappear forever. Any suggestions? Buy a couple of cases of it and keep replenishing your stock regularly, so that you always have several months' supply in the house.

"I'm Not Losing Any More"

Question:

I felt so good when I was losing weight on your method. For several months, I was losing three or four pounds a month. But suddenly I've stopped losing. I still have twenty-five pounds to go and I feel discouraged.

Answer:

It may be reassuring to you that most people reach such plateaus once in a while. They are to be expected.

You may be focusing too much on weight loss or on the rate of loss. This tends to create tension and guilt feelings whenever you eat high-calorie foods — all of which infringes on your food freedom. See if you can once again focus on what is humming to you; concentrate on the pleasure aspect of food. It might help to go over some of the awareness exercises. If you've not been keeping a journal, you might begin one now to record your moods and food preferences. This can sharpen your insights.

"I'm Hungry but Nothing Hums"

Question: Sometimes when I actually feel hunger pangs and try to tune in to what is humming, I draw a blank. What should I do?

Answer: Satisfy your physiological hunger with just a few bites of almost any food. Eat only until the hunger pangs that accompany true physiological hunger stop. A small amount of food generally suffices — for instance, half a banana. If you experience no pangs, and don't know what hums to you, chances are the answer is "nothing." A good rule is that if you have to ask, then you probably don't have anything humming.

Going on a Chocolate-Candy Jag

Question: Ever since being in your workshop I've lost weight, but I eat almost a whole box of candy on some days. When this happens, I feel satisfied and don't eat anything else on those days. Is this O.K.?

Answer: Yes.

How to Get Taken Care of

Question: The kind of food I eat is not as important to me as having someone take care of me by cooking my meals. What I really wish is that (I can't afford it, but I really wish) someone would prepare everything and then serve it to me. Sometimes I don't even want the bother of making choices. Can you suggest a way out for me?

Answer: If you can find a friend who has similar feelings you could trade off being each other's guest at dinner.

Your feeling is a valid and understandable response. This happens especially to women who have spent most of their lives feeding and serving and caring for others, including adult men. It's very understandable that someone would yearn for a period of time when they need no longer think about food-gathering or food-preparation.

"She Said I Tempted Her"

Question: We gave a cocktail party last weekend and I had fun making a lot of different hors d'oeuvres, ones that I really love. But an old friend of mine was upset because she said she had counted on my serving nonfattening things, and here I was tempting her with all these high-calorie goodies. I didn't know what to say.

Answer: That's her problem, not yours. You can't solve the eating problems of other adults. Every person has to assume responsibility for their own eating. Tell your friend you wouldn't be offended if she brought her own low-calorie snacks next time she comes to your house.

"I Don't Want to Get Thin"

Question: The more I think about it, the more I feel I really don't want to get thin right now. I think I want to avoid dating and sex for a while and get my head together. I wonder if I'm freaky, or does that happen to other people, too?

Answer: It does. Not being thin may serve a definite purpose in your life right now. If it does, it makes psychological sense to stay overweight. A goal might be to be able to say "yes" or "no" to sex without using your body weight as the method of avoiding the issue.

Special Events and Dining Out

Question: Sometimes going out to dinner at a fine restaurant isn't what I really feel like, but I do want a sense of something special. In the town where my husband and I live, going out to dinner seems almost the only "special" thing to do. Any suggestions?

Answer: I personally (Lil) have found that there's a special feeling of luxury in just spending some money, and it doesn't have to be at a restaurant. Instead, it can be anything that feels immediate and seems wasteful. My favorite splurge is buying lovely flowers, and the ultimate in luxury is to buy the perfect vase at the flower shop to go with exactly those length flowers. What ways of doing something special would please you?

The Fourteen-Year-Old Who Sneaks Candy

Question: My fourteen-year-old son uses his lunch and allowance money to buy candy and cookies. How can I stop him?

Answer: You can't. However, you might consider this: Children who have full opportunity *and* freedom to eat sweets at home don't have to sneak candy. The child rebels if he doesn't have this opportunity and feels deprived of sweets. Then he will obtain them whenever and wherever he can.

Please note that we said "opportunity *and* freedom to eat sweets at home." A friend of ours complained that her children were still making clandestine trips to the ice cream store and buying candy on the sly even after she offered to buy each daughter her own box of candy and her own bag of cookies.

"They didn't really want me to," she said in puzzlement. It turned out that the girls had no trust in their mother's change of heart about candies. From the way she approached the whole subject and the way she continued to handle other tension-producing eating occasions such as family dessert ("Finish your meat loaf first"), they couldn't believe that they would not be censured, even with their own bag of candy.

Before any change could occur, she had to bridge the credibility gap.

Keep that in mind and also the fact that, ultimately, all children assume full responsibility for their bodies and their own eating. At age fourteen, that time is here for your son.

"I Had Freed My Body"

Question: In your follow-up questionnaire you ask, "Have there been any changes in any aspect of your life that you attribute to the workshop experience?" I've noticed that I've been enjoying sex more during the past two months. Have you ever heard this from anyone else?

Answer: Yes. Here is an example of how guilt feelings about the way one's body is used with respect to food can spill over into a person's total life!

In a workshop we conducted last year, one of the participants, Marian, described herself as a nut freak. As she drove to and from work along the endless Los Angeles freeways, she kept a bag or small can of peanuts next to her and devoured them during the first thirty minutes of driving. She often tried to fool herself by keeping the nuts in the glove compartment or even putting them out of reach in the trunk. But she found that efforts to maneuver herself were useless. She would pull off the road onto the shoulder, go back to the trunk, grab a handful of nuts, put the can back in the trunk, and return to her driving. She would do this several times, each time feeling stupid and angry at herself.

During the workshop she developed insight into how she was using food and realized the importance of experiencing her previously "sinful" or "illicit" foods.

Sunday morning when she came into the workshop group, she seemed to be floating about six inches off the floor, her face glowing. Several people asked her what had happened and she then explained: "I've been married for almost two years, and last night when my husband made love to me I had my first orgasm!" She also described how she had bought a three--pound can of nuts and kept it right next to her in the car, with the top off, after leaving the workshop Saturday. To her surprise, she ate only a few handfuls instead of the usual pound.

She put it succinctly: "Responding freely to my body in one way seems to have changed how I responded in other ways. I had freed my body."

The fact that she felt less self-hatred may also have helped her to feel that she deserved pleasure in food or otherwise.

A Word for the Uninitiated

Question: Any ideas for a quick, witty retort when people
             ask me what sort of a goofy diet I'm on now?
Answer: How about saying it's a "Pleasure Diet"!

But Does It Really Work?

Question: Your method sounds too good to be true. Does it
             really work?
Answer: Yes. After working with more than two thousand
             people over the past seventeen years, I can state
             that the overwhelming majority have lost weight
             permanently.

             However, during the past eighteen months
             we have made a systematic follow-up by ques-
             tionnaire of nearly five hundred people who
             came to our Institute workshops. The results
             show that nearly 35 percent have lost weight
             through our approach of pleasure-eating. This is
             in sharp contrast to the 2 percent success rate
             accomplished by the traditional method of diet
             and pills. Another 35 percent of the people we
             surveyed have achieved easy maintenance of
             their current weight: They are liberated eaters
             who have discarded all diets!

             The remaining group (about 30 percent)
             have had difficulty in accepting or applying our
             system and have continued on with their

roller-coaster style of losing and gaining, dieting and hinging.

On follow-up, we find that almost all (nearly 95 percent) of those we worked with are spending less energy fighting food, have changed their concept of eating, and suffer much less from self-hatred. For the first time in years, they are actually enjoying food — and life.

What About Guarantees?

Question.   Is your method guaranteed to lose weight?
Answer: No ethical psychologist, physician or lawyer, or any other professional guarantees results. This would be contrary to the code of ethical behavior of all established professions. Quacks, frauds and some patent medicine companies do this because there is usually no way to hold them to their promises. Some weight salons and similar establishments offer "money-back guarantees," knowing full well that most people are too embarrassed by failure or too intimidated to ask for the return of their money.

What honest professionals offer is advice, based on their training, experience and knowledge, in an effort to help you. Human behavior is so complicated, and one's weight is affected by so many variables, that a guarantee for any individual is impossible. But liberated eating has helped thousands of people we've worked with, and seems to be used by millions of thin people who pleasure themselves with food without being aware that they are, in fact, "liberated eaters."

We want to thank you for purchasing this book. Our writers and creative team took pride in creating this book, and we have tried to make it as enjoyable as possible.

We would love to hear from you, kindly leave a review if you enjoyed this book so we can do more. Your reviews on our books are highly appreciated. Also, if you have any comments or suggestions, you may reach us at

info@contentarcade.com

Regards,
Content Arcade Publishing Team